Nancy Phelan is a Sydney writer, photographer and traveller. She has been a serious student of yoga for many years and was trained as a teacher by Michael Volin, who founded the first yoga school in Australia. Now associated with this school, Nancy Phelan has had a wide experience with pupils of all ages. Besides *Yoga Over Forty*, written with Michael Volin, she is the author of a novel and two travel books.

Beginners Guide to Yoga

NANCY PHELAN

SPHERE BOOKS LIMITED
30/32 Gray's Inn Road, London WC1X 8JL

First published in Great Britain by
Pelham Books Ltd 1973
Copyright © Nancy Phelan 1973
Published by Sphere Books 1976

TRADE MARK

Set in Photon Baskerville

Printed in Great Britain by
C. Nicholls & Company Ltd
The Philips Park Press, Manchester

CONTENTS

HOW TO USE THIS BOOK   Page 9

CHAPTER ONE   FACTS ABOUT YOGA   11
What yoga is . . . Its background and aims . . . There is more than one kind of yoga . . . *Hatha* (physical) yoga in the West . . . Questions asked by beginners . . . What is the right age to start . . . How yoga helps, mentally and physically . . . Learning from a book . . . Practising at home . . . What you need . . . What to wear . . . Spiritual aspects . . . Higher stages of training.

CHAPTER TWO   HOW YOGA WORKS   22
A balanced attitude . . . Ascetic yogis . . . Delaying old age . . . How and why it is done . . . Fighting central gravity and physical deterioration . . . The five groups of *asanas* in this book . . . Yoga Breathing . . . *Prana* . . . Maintaining vital energy . . . How to breathe correctly . . . Yoga breathing in daily life . . . Calming the emotions . . . The power of breath.

CHAPTER THREE   PRACTISING AT HOME   31
How long should practice last? . . . How to fit it into a busy life . . . How to practise . . . The importance of relaxation . . . Sequence of instruction outlined . . . Learning to arrange your own practice sequence . . . Cautions and Prohibitions . . . Stiffness . . . Mental attitude.

CHAPTER FOUR   *HATHA* YOGA IN THE FORM OF A
LESSON   36
Savasana – Pose of Complete Rest
... Limbering up ... Pacifying Breaths ...
Recharging Cycle ... Cleansing Breath
... Preliminary Exercises for different
parts of the body ... Pose of an Eagle ...
Stomach Contractions: *Uddiyana* (Stand-
ing) ... *Nauli* ... Shoulderstand ... Half-
Shoulderstand ... Pose of Tranquillity
... Balancing Shoulderstand ... Modi-
fied Fish Pose ... Pose of a Cobra ...
Pose of a Locust ... Bow Pose ... Easy
Pose ... Mental Exercise: Creating a
Flower ... Head and Neck Exercises ...
Eye Exercises ... Arch Gesture and
Variations ... Pose of a Star ... Modified
Splits Pose ... Head-to-Knee Pose
(Sitting) ... Angular Pose ... Pose of an
Archer ... Sideways Swing ... Spinal
Twist ... Pose of a Cat ... Supine Pelvic
Pose ... Pose of a Child ... Pose of a Bird
... *Savasana* ... Exercises to restore
circulation   (Shaking   limbs)   ...
Headstand.

CHAPTER FIVE   FURTHER PRACTICE   74
Additional Breathing Cycles: Recharging;
Pacifying; Purifying ... Additional exer-
cises for back, chest, waist, stomach, hips,
feet and legs ... To increase height and
improve posture ... The Magic of Slow
Movements ... Exercises for facial
muscles ... Additional *asanas*: Diamond
Pose ... Pose of a Frog ... Pose of a
Hero ... Free Pose ... Pose of an Adept
... Half-Lotus Pose ... Lotus Position
... *Advasana* ... Pose of a Hare ... Head-
to-Knee Pose (Standing) ... Pose of a
Plough ... Half-Locust Pose ... Pose of

an Archer – Variation . . . Little Twist . . .
Pose of a Camel . . . Half-Wheel Pose . . .
Surya Namaskar – Greeting to the Rising
Sun . . . Pose of a Lion . . . Head of a Cow
Pose . . . Pose of a Tree . . . Digestive
Cycle . . . *Uddiyana* (Sitting) . . . Knees-
to-Stomach Pose . . . Solar Plexus Pose
. . . Pose of a Raven . . . Pose of Eight
Curves . . . Inverted Bird Pose or Half-
Headstand.

CHAPTER SIX   MENTAL TRAINING   105
Higher and lower meditation . . . Pre-
liminaries to meditation . . . Development
of Concentration . . . Inversion of the
Mind's Eye . . . Development of Inner
Strength . . . Development of Will-Power
. . . Overcoming Temptation . . . I am
Stronger than Fear . . . The Seven Fears
. . . I am Master of Myself . . . Concentra-
tion on Universal Goodness . . . Con-
centration on the Object of Love and
Devotion . . . Protective Cocoon . . . With-
drawal from External Influences . . .
Meditation on the Day to Come and on
the Day just Past.

CHAPTER SEVEN   THE METHOD PLUS YOURSELF   113
The human body . . . joints . . . digestive
and eliminative systems . . . respiration
. . . nerves . . . glands . . . Hygiene . . .
Purification . . . Care of Teeth . . . Hair
. . . Eyes . . . Inner cleanliness . . . Weight
. . . Posture . . . Rest and Relaxation . . .
Sleep.

CHAPTER EIGHT   YOGA AND DIET   131
Improved attitude to diet . . . The yoga
diet . . . Principles for guidance: Selectivity, Moderation and Mastication . . .

Vegetarianism ... Meatless meals ... Making your own yoghurt ... Fasting ... Seasonal Purification ... Tobacco ... Alcohol ... Drugs.

CHAPTER NINE   MORE ABOUT YOGA   142
The three main kinds of yogis: Ascetic, Tantric and Householder ... The higher yogas: *Rajah* ... *Jnani* ... *Kundalini* ... *Kundalini* and the *Cakras* ... *Samadhi* ... *Bhakti* yoga ... *Karma* Yoga ... The life of Right Action ... Non-attachment ... great *Karma* yogis ... *Karma* and Re-incarnation ... *Hatha* yoga ... The Eight Steps of *Hatha* Yoga ... *Samadhi* attained through yoga and through L.S.D.

CHAPTER TEN   PRACTICE GUIDE   152
Twenty-two Reminders for Beginners ... Suggested routines for varying amounts of practice time, from minimum to un-limited ... Suggested practice sequences, one for each day of the week.

For Further Reading   159

Appendix: *To help overcome smoking habit*   160

ILLUSTRATIONS

Over ninety instructional photographs in the text give step-by-step guidance on the *asanas* of *Hatha* yoga. We ac-knowledge with thanks permission from *Woman's World* (Australia) to reproduce the following photographs: 11B, 14B, 17A–D, 22A–D, 24C–F, 37, 42A+B, 50A–D, 56A–C.

HOW TO USE THIS BOOK

Although this book is written on the assumption that the reader is a beginner, it could also be used by more experienced students for practice at home. The main section is arranged in the form of an illustrated lesson. The order in which the exercises and *asanas* (bodily positions) are grouped is the carefully-thought-out sequence of instruction used by Michael Volin in his school of *Hatha* yoga. It is based on years of knowledge and teaching experience in East and West and has proved suitable and successful with Western students.

Due to entirely different conditions and ways of life, *Hatha* yoga in the West cannot be taught exactly as in an Eastern *ashram*, where the disciple lives constantly with his teacher; but Michael Volin's aim has always been to retain the true message of yoga while adapting the method of training to Western life, and apart from a few inevitable modifications the traditional basic truth of the teaching is unchanged.

Instructions have been set out as simply as possible to make them easy to follow while practising, but before attempting the lesson *read through the whole book several times*. Don't just prop it up and try to follow directions as though making a new kind of cake. This is particularly important if you know nothing of yoga, or if you are trying to teach yourself. You must have a clear general picture of what you are doing and why, not only for your own interest but to avoid possible misinterpretation.

All the *asanas* in the book could not be included in one lesson, but there are certain poses which should be practised each time for tonic and strengthening effects. These are marked ★. Other poses, exercises and breathing cycles not so marked could be varied from time to time.

Regard your practice as a treatment for your body, not as a course to be mastered as quickly as possible so you can move on to something else. Yoga is too good and too valuable to be approached in this spirit.

This *Beginner's Guide* is based on an earlier book by Michael Volin and Nancy Phelan, published in Australia as *Essence of Yoga* and in the United States as *The Spirit and Practice of Yoga*, but not previously published in the U.K. The original text has been completely revised, enlarged, brought up to date and adapted for the use of beginners. Advanced *asanas* have been replaced by more of the simpler poses, and extra chapters have been added.

In a book of this kind, which is in fact a lesson, some repetition is inevitable and necessary. It not only helps the student to remember, it makes for easier reference. Though the *asanas* in Chapter Four are given as a continuing sequence, each one may be referred to separately without turning to other pages for information on cautions, purpose, etc.

Readers acquainted with other books by Michael Volin and myself may find some familiar material in this one, but where such material is also important for beginners it has been necessary to include it. On the other hand every effort has been made to ensure that nothing is too difficult for a beginner and to avoid taking for granted any previous knowledge. In this I have consulted beginners among my own students, and to them I express my gratitude.

My main debt, of course, is to Michael Volin, who was not only the originator of the earlier book but who, as my teacher, introduced me to a practice and philosophy that has become part of my life.

NANCY PHELAN
Sydney 1972

Chapter One

FACTS ABOUT YOGA

Though people all over the world are now happily practising yoga, misconceptions still persist. To some it is just another form of physical jerks, to others an odd hippie cult that could possibly conflict with religious beliefs. Even the most enthusiastic devotees of *Hatha* (physical) yoga do not always realise exactly what is behind their training or suspect the fascinating possibilities that it can open up.

Hatha yoga, the oldest existing physical culture system in the world, is a scientific combination of exercise and breathing, but it is also a profound philosophy, one that equips us to face life, overcome defeats, accept the inevitable and endure what may seem unendurable. It is a way of living, of thinking; an inward journey of endless discovery that opens up the individual self and brings out the best from those who practise it.

It is neither a weird cult nor a religion. It has no priests or dogma, nor does it affect any personal beliefs, except perhaps to intensify and deepen the capacity for religious experience. Yoga classes are often held in church halls or organised by church groups, and one frequently hears people say that they have become better Christians because yoga has made them more patient, understanding and compassionate. It is practised by believers of many faiths in many parts of the world.

Its aim is universal: peace and serenity through *yoga* or union with God, (also known as Liberation, Identification, Self-Realisation). The name comes from the ancient language of India, the Sanscrit root *yuj* – to join or yoke, and has a dual significance. Physically, it refers to the special method of breathing, while its deeper meaning is the underlying spiritual purpose.

Yoga is the goal and also the name of the way by which we try to reach it. A man who practises *yoga* is a *yogi*, a woman is called a *yogini*. A *guru* is the teacher or spiritual guide of a yogi. His name means 'One who dispels darkness'. In the west, where yoga teachers are less often spiritual guides, 'Instructor' is a more suitable term. A great teacher, like Gandhi, is a *mahatma*.

Gurus may live isolated in caves, or in *ashrams* (hermitages) with their disciples. *Ashrams* vary from the most primitive to peaceful retreats with beautiful gardens and sometimes up-to-date equipment. One much-publicised establishment has air-conditioned meditation cells for those who are affected by the heat of India. This is agreeable but hardly in the true yogic tradition.

A number of *ashrams* in India take western students for study and instruction. In the East, the serious student, or *chela*, lives constantly with his *guru*, who watches over every step of his training and development. It is believed that knowledge should only be passed on to those who are ready for it and sometimes a *chela* has great difficulty finding his *guru*. He may have to search for years, for unlike the West, where people are usually taught in classes and sometimes change their teachers, or even learn from several at the same time, the traditional relationship between *guru* and disciple is far more personal; they must be completely in tune with each other in every way, a spiritual father-and-son relationship. It is said that when the pupil is ready the teacher appears.

In India, which has always been a highly spiritual country, it is not at all uncommon for successful professional people or businessmen, having reached middle age, to provide for their families and go off to seek a *guru* and devote the rest of their lives to spiritual training and preparation for death. Though few Western householders can do this, they could go a considerable way along the path while still living out in the world.

Thousands of people now use the physical training of yoga purely for health and beauty. There is nothing wrong in this; many weak, tired and discouraged men and women have been helped by it and by the friendships they have formed through attending classes; but it is not the whole of yoga. Exercises alone will not comfort the lonely nor give an all-absorbing purpose to a sad or empty life.

Yoga is one of India's six great philosophies. It is said to have been revealed to men by the god Siva himself. We do not know its age, only that it goes back thousands of years and that it is mentioned in the Vedas, India's sacred scriptures. Archeologists excavating in the most ancient parts of the Indus Valley have discovered figures of men in yogic poses. Some of these may be seen in museums, not only in India but also in England, France, Germany and the U.S.A.

About the third century, some scholars say earlier, the sage Patanjali collected and codified a number of ancient yoga *sutras* (aphorisms), forming one of the great classical yoga texts. It is known as the *Yoga Darshana* and Patanjali himself is often called the Father of Yoga.

It is not always realised that there is more than one kind of yoga or yogic path. From earliest times the people of India have been much concerned with spiritual development, but since men vary, and what suits one may not suit another, a number of yogas or spiritual paths evolved through the centuries. There is one for each type, each need – a path of action; of contemplation; of intense mental discipline; of physical strength; of knowledge; of religious worship – but whatever the path, the ultimate goal is the same: union of the individual soul with the soul of the universe, the realization that the ego-Self is only part of the Universal Self, or God.

People follow the path that most appeals to them, that they are best suited for. For Western householders the most suitable are *Hatha* yoga, the path of bodily strength and control; *Karma* yoga, the path of right action; and *Bhakti* yoga, the path of love and devotion, of religious worship. It often happens that the three are mixed; for instance, a man or woman who does *Hatha* yoga to keep fit, who always tries to be helpful and kind, who is not obsessed with material possessions or enslaved by greed and ambition, and who is also sincerely religious, is following all three paths, even though he or she has never heard their names.

Beginners sometimes ask if they should become vegetarian and celibate in order to practise yoga, if they are expected to give away everything and live like a monk. There is no need for extreme measures in the case of the average student; it is possible to be a sincere follower of yoga while living a normal family life.*

On the other hand, a yogi who has dedicated himself to one of the ascetic paths must renounce the world, retire to an *ashram* or forest cave, alone or with his teacher, observing celibacy and a very austere diet. He must practise arduous purifications; he owns nothing, his whole life and all his energies are devoted to attaining yoga or Self-Realisation. The reasons for his strict disciplines, which are explained further in Chapter Nine, are not likely to concern the ordinary Western student. For him, the main requirements are moderation in everything and a genuine desire for yoga and to live a good life. He need not become vegetarian if it does not suit him, though after some time of practising yoga the desire for meat may decrease, and he is not obliged to give up sex. In fact, *Hatha* yoga is known to be beneficial to sex life through its effect on the glands and through raising the general standard of health. There is no preaching or proselytising; only the example, if one wishes to reach the goal. For those who are not interested in the spiritual path there is no compulsion to follow it.

Hatha yoga, the path best known in the West, and the main subject of this book, brings the body to its highest stage of perfection and under complete control of the mind. The training is built round a nucleus of 84 *asanas* or bodily positions, and practice brings strength, grace and suppleness. It tones up the glands and internal organs, improves the circulation, regulates weight, delays ageing – an important part of yoga – increases vital energy and teaches the art of relaxation. All these benefits react on the mind and personality. When the body is in perfect working order the outlook is cheerful and optimistic; when the nerves are calm and relaxed the attitude is more philosophical towards setbacks. There are also mental exercises to develop character, inner strength, moral courage and concentration, and for those who desire it, the practice of meditation.

*Apart from reasons of purification, the yogi is a vegetarian because he does not wish to take life.

A question frequently asked is, 'Am I too old· to start? What is the right age?' Though with most things it is always good to start young there is really no 'right age' for yoga. Its peaceful philosophy has something for everyone, no matter what age or physical condition. Those who cannot do the physical practice could learn to relax tension and increase their energy through improved breathing; to meditate, to make the journey into themselves. In fact, older people usually make better students; they have a more mature attitude, a deeper understanding and experience of life which gives greater patience and perseverence.

Six is the traditional starting age for children. Sometimes toddlers who come to class with their mothers like to try the *asanas*, and though they usually accomplish them easily, since their joints are so flexible, they should not be allowed to try anything that might adversely affect growing bones; for instance they should not do the Headstand while the bones of the skull are still soft, and even when older the neck is not always strong enough to take the weight of the body in this pose, or the strain of the Plough and the Choking Pose. But no one is too young to be taught correct breathing and healthy living habits.

Middle-aged beginners are sometimes unnecessarily depressed about stiffness, yet youth is no guarantee of suppleness. Teenagers are often extremely stiff, for many young people take almost no exercise and their bodies have no chance to limber up. They rarely walk, they spend most of their lives sitting, in cars, in offices, at desks, watching television. They do not exert themselves in housework or gardening and those who play games often develop only certain sets of muscles without much benefit to the rest. Swimming and ballet dancing, which exercise most of the body, are the main exceptions.

Though younger students may start with enthusiasm they cannot always stay the distance. They dislike work and discipline and may grow bored if success does not come quickly. In *Hatha* yoga, physical facility is not always an advantage; those who do things too easily do not always value them or have the patience and humility needed for true progress. They miss the real significance of the training.

Sometimes young students set out to master as many *asanas* as fast as they can; one hears them listing their achievements in a way that reveals complete lack of understanding of even the physical side of yoga. It is the repeated attempt, the practice, the constant exercising of muscles and joints, the continual challenge of failure and obstacles to be overcome that develop not only body but character and will-power. Older people who have tenacity and a desire to succeed have nothing to fear from the young.

Though too much confidence may be an obstacle, not enough is just as bad. Adults who become too easily discouraged by the physical feats of others must learn to approach yoga in a different spirit. For them, the purpose is not the same as for the young; they should not worry about spectacular poses but concentrate on *asanas* and techniques most applicable to themselves, most needed to keep their bodies slim and agile, to delay ageing and prolong the creative part of life. They should spend more time on relaxation and recharging with vital energy, which is particularly important for women going through the menopause and for overweight businessmen with high blood pressure. They could also turn to inner development, to mental exercises or to meditation and the pursuit of Self-Realisation. This brings serenity and a philosophical attitude to the last years of life, even towards death.

Would-be beginners sometimes say they would like to watch a lesson before they start, 'to see what it's like.' This could be compared to expecting to taste an apple by watching someone else eat it. No one can show you how yoga feels, you must do the *asanas* yourself. Others admit tentatively that they want to see if they could do it before starting. They are really inviting defeat, for they often decide it all looks so hard they can never bring themselves to try. They develop an inferiority complex and slink away, beaten before they start. Men and women who have let themselves go and not exercised properly for many years could find it unnerving to see youthful-looking grandmothers standing on their heads. They might even get the impression that such students have been training for most of their lives, when in fact these supple, graceful bodies were stiff and shapeless not long before.

Occasionally beginners are persuaded to come to class by a determined and enthusiastic friend, or sent by a doctor or psychiatrist. Once they have made the effort to start there are few who do not continue. There may be a little cheerful groaning at first but more often it is an air of pleased surprise and eagerness for the next lesson. Older people, who expected to feel self-conscious among young students, find that no one is taking any notice of them, that each pupil is completely absorbed in his or her own activities; and to their relief and astonishment they are not at all stiff next day. This is due to the gentle and leisurely pace of the movements.

In the classical texts one may find very strange claims made for the power of yoga. It is said to cure all sorts of complaints, even to overcome death. These statements are often symbolical; for instance, overcoming death does not necessarily mean eternal life in this body but the release of the perfected spirit after *karma* has been worked out (see page 144, for *karma*).

Extravagant and unreasonable claims are also made by modern Western enthusiasts, but though yoga is not a miracle cure-all it does indeed correct and improve many physical conditions and greatly help in times of emotional and mental stress. It is not yoga alone that solves the problems; it is yoga *plus* yourself. It changes you, not the situation; it is always *you* who must cope but it is yoga that gives you the extra strength, the better balance, the calmness, the higher mental development needed to find your way. It is no instant remedy; like everything else worthwhile it demands work and perseverence. It does for you whatever you do for it, and gives back according to what you put into it.

Yoga should always be kept a personal affair, studied and practised for your own physical, mental and spiritual development. It should not be regarded purely as a means of material gain or of earning a living. It should never be subjected to cheapening promotion or brought down to a lower level to attract followers.

Some of the higher teachings are kept secret; the texts are

obscure and incomplete because it is believed that they lose their power if exposed to the public. This obscurity also prevents the ignorant and uninitiated from tampering with practices that could be dangerous for unprepared bodies and minds.

There are no grounds for fears that physical yoga gives bulging muscles. The body becomes stronger, firmer and more flexible, but development is neither unbalanced nor exaggerated because of the scientific system of exercise, and because of the action of the glands.

New pupils frequently ask how long it takes to learn the poses, or what is the length of a course. To answer the first of these questions, progress is entirely individual. A few are naturally supple but for most, practice is essential; the more you loosen up the body the more easily you will do the *asanas*, but there should never be any haste or anxiety. Yoga is non-competitive and slowness in learning is not important, so long as you keep trying.

As for the length of a so-called course, in true yoga there is no such thing. Learning is a continuing process and one either gives up or goes on for life. In the west, sometimes for convenience, teachers may divide the year into terms, but it is not traditional practice; nor is the growing tendency to offer diplomas at the end of a certain period. This prevails among those who believe that yoga, like trimming hats or making lampshades, could be mastered in a reasonable time and used as a means of making money. It has been encouraged by the increasing popularity of this philosophy, and has resulted in a great proliferation of teachers of varying competence.

It is often asked if yoga can be learnt from a book, and for those who live in areas where there is no teacher this may be the only way. In the East, instruction has always been by mouth-to-ear, from *guru* to *chela*, and even in the West personal tuition is preferred. *Hatha* yoga deals with the delicate mechanisms of the human body, the circulation, nervous systems, glands and internal organs and misinterpreted instructions could cause imbalance or injury.

18

But if you sincerely want to learn and cannot get a teacher, a good book is better than nothing, if used with care and commonsense. It is advisable to have a medical check-up first, in case there is some unsuspected condition like high bloodpressure or a spinal disc weakness, in which case certain poses should not be attempted till the condition has improved. This advice applies to all students, not only those who hope to teach themselves. If you have any doubts at all about your health, or if you are pregnant, ask your doctor's advice. Most medical men are now familiar with yoga and generally approve of it.

There is a considerable literature, both scholarly and popular, on *Hatha* yoga and it should be possible to get a really reliable book, written by an experienced teacher. Read all instructions with full attention and do not try anything until you are sure you have understood them. Proceed slowly and cautiously, never straining yourself in any way or forcing the body into poses it is not ready for. Muscles and ligaments are like elastic; they may be stretched by gentle persuasion but might snap back and tear if pulled too suddenly or violently. Such damage is not only painful but could put you out of action for months.

Always rest and relax between the *asanas*, and remember that pain is a stop signal, a warning to give up and try again next time. If it persists, consult a doctor.

When cautions and prohibitions are given they must be observed. Some poses are absolutely forbidden in certain conditions and ignoring the warnings could lead to harm. These warnings are repeated throughout this book; they cannot be over-emphasised, for people continue to try and teach themselves too advanced or unsuitable techniques, and teachers continue to receive appeals for help from those who have injured themselves in the process.

Many beginners who come to class find they also need a book for use when practising at home. This is particularly noticeable when they have joined a group of more advanced students and are having difficulty trying to keep up. A book helps them to understand details that are already known to the others and which may otherwise never become quite clarified.

19

Very little equipment is needed for yoga practice; just enough room to lie down and exercise in, and a rug or a mat or a piece of foam rubber. The traditional yogi's seat is of grass and antelope skin.

Ballet tights and leotards for women are very comfortable and popular, and not too expensive, but though they certainly give the most freedom they are by no means obligatory. Shirt and shorts with bare legs, swimming costumes, tights and a sweater could be used, even an athlete's track suit. Ordinary slacks are usually too constricting for the legs.

Men wear trunks, or shorts, with or without a shirt or sweater.

There are students who would like to study the spiritual aspects of yoga but who fear that they are not intellectual or highly-educated enough. This idea is wrong. Though certain paths are more suitable for intellectuals, intellect alone never achieved yoga. The mind is only a tool – a vital one in getting us through life – but it is not everything. There is something more important, the mysterious essence, the indestructible spark that raises man above the animals and which we call the soul. It has nothing to do with intellect; it functions not through the mind but through intuition, providing a direct contact with the Supreme Spirit. This is why highly spiritual people and great saints have sometimes been simple and quite uneducated in the formal sense. The Upanishads, the sacred scriptures of India, tell us that Self-Realisation – yoga – will never be attained through study of the scriptures or intellect or great learning, but only by he who longs for it; and that all the many forms of philosophy, arguments, grammatical rules are traps to catch the intellect and lead it astray from true knowledge.

Other students sometimes ask if yoga is connected with magic; they have heard of yogis being buried alive or performing strange feats. Yoga teaches that we are all part of the universe; that our bodies and the natural world round us are manifestations of the same force, and that with knowledge and training man could learn to control this force, both within his own physical frame and beyond it. At a certain stage of advancement a yogi may develop exceptional powers of this kind. It is said that we are all born with them in a latent form but that they never develop because of ignorance, wrong ways of living and lack of training. (Many Western mystics possessed them in various degrees ... powers of levitation, clairvoyance, telepathy).

These powers, or *siddhis*, are not magic; they come from extraordinary understanding and control of natural laws and the true yogi recognises them for what they are. He knows that they are incidental to his progress, marking a stage of development, and that they could be a trap to impede further spiritual progress. Some yogis do become trapped; they use their psychic powers to make money, or display them to impress disciples. India is full of such people; they vary from roadside performers to wealthy *gurus* with thousands of trusting followers. These are not true yogis, no matter how great their knowledge and power.

Though sometimes a yogi, in the interests of science, may submit himself to medical tests, the real holy man does not display himself; he is usually very hard to find, living alone, or perhaps with a disciple, in the forest or a cave in the Himalayas, dedicated and absorbed in his search for God.

Chapter Two

HOW YOGA WORKS

In their eagerness to persuade the public that *Hatha* yoga is not a weird oriental cult some people have gone too far in the opposite direction, presenting it as no more than a means of staying young and beautiful. It is now included in courses at charm schools and used to promote anything from ballet tights to the products of health food shops; other enthusiasts regard it as a training for circus-like contortions. But the intelligent student must aim for a balance, keeping the body active and healthy while developing mind and spirit.

Though *Hatha* yoga is so ancient, it is completely scientific and logical. Every gesture has a purpose, to improve, develop or strengthen, but all are designed ultimately to bring stillness of mind.

A serious disciple seeking liberation of the spirit (*moksa*) will spend much of his time in meditation and breathing techniques in one or other of the sitting poses. Regular practice of the *asanas* not only gives the necessary strength and endurance for this demanding discipline but also provides healthy and much-needed exercise in what would be otherwise a very sedentary life.

Some of the more primitive ascetic yogis believe that liberation of the spirit comes through mortifying the flesh. One sees them in India, face and body daubed with mud or cow dung, matted hair, long dirty nails and equally dirty garments or perhaps no clothes at all. The true *Hatha* yogi regards his body as the temple of the living spirit; he keeps it clean outside and purified within, strong, and in the best working order.

An important aim of *Hatha* yoga is to delay the process of ageing, to prolong the creative part of life. The human body matures much more quickly than the mind; a man may be fully grown but still mentally and emotionally immature. By the time his mind has developed his body is usually starting to deteriorate. The yoga ideal is a mature mind in a young and vigorous body; therefore age is held back to give the mind time to catch up, to allow man to acquire wisdom while still enjoying health, strength and vitality. Since yoga teaches that the body does not finish growing till the age of thirty-three, the years from fifty-five to seventy-five are regarded as the prime of life.

The desired effects are obtained by careful working on joints, muscles, circulation, digestive and eliminative systems, nerves and glands. Certain *asanas* are designed to keep the joints supple, to limber up the spine; others concentrate on the endocrinal glands, on purifying the bloodstream, on redirecting the circulation, sending it to parts of the body starved of arterial blood. There are raised poses to help retain lightness and buoyancy and preserve relative strength; balancing poses for physical and mental equilibrium; abdominal contractions to tone up the internal organs. There are also exercises for eyes, neck and face muscles.

Correct respiration increases the vital energy, improved intake of oxygen purifies the bloodstream and certain breathing techniques relax nervous tension. Inverting the body, turning it upside-down, is a very important part of practice. The inverted poses work on the metabolic processes, regulating and toning-up the glands, and at the same time help the body resist the downward pull of gravity, which is a powerful contributor to physical ageing.

We tend to forget or ignore the fact that the strong force which holds us to the earth is also pulling us down all our lives. Only will-power keeps us upright; if we faint or lose consciousness we fall; when we are tired or ill or resistance is lowered in any way we want to lie down. As people grow older, if their vital energy has diminished, they offer less and less resistance to central gravity; they sit about more, they even take to their beds and become bedridden.

The constant pull shows in sick, tired and ageing faces, in dejected downward lines, sagging muscles, fallen arches, dropped organs. Reversing the body not only resists the pull of gravity but helps to correct such displacements. This method, combined with yoga breathing to increase vital energy, is one of our greatest defences against old age.

Maintaining suppleness of joints, and particularly the spine, is also important in holding back ageing. (It is said in yoga that old age begins with stiffening of the backbone). The spine is all-important in training, not only because it contains the spinal cord, a main point of focus in higher practices, but because the general condition of the whole body depends on a healthy spine. Nerves go out from the spinal cord to every part and if they are neglected and deprived of arterial blood they will degenerate. When the spine is properly exercised the circulation of blood to the roots of the spinal nerves increases and keeps them healthy (see Chapter Seven).

The poses in this book could be divided into five groups:

SITTING POSES, used mainly for meditation, breathing techniques, neck and eye exercises: Easy Pose; Pose of an Adept; Free Pose; Half-Lotus; Lotus Position; Pose of a Hero; Pose of a Frog; Head of a Cow Pose; Diamond Pose; Pose of a Lion.

INVERTED POSES, for the metabolical processes, the endocrinal glands: Shoulderstand; Half-shoulderstand: Pose of Tranquillity; Balancing Shoulderstand; Headstand and Half-headstand (or Inverted Bird).

STRETCHING CYCLE, for preserving suppleness in spine and joints, arresting and preventing calcification: Arch Gesture and Variations; Head-to-Knee Pose, in sitting and standing position; Pose of a Plough; Choking Pose; Sideways Swing; Pose of an Archer; Spinal Twist; Little Twist; Pose of a Star; Cobra; Bow Pose; Locust; Supine Pelvic; Camel Pose; Pose of a Cat; Half-Locust Pose.

RAISED POSES, to preserve physical lightness and buoyancy: Pose of a Bird; Pose of a Raven; Pose of Eight Curves.

VARIOUS POSES AND TECHNIQUES: Abdominal contractions for digestive and eliminative systems: *Uddiyana; Nauli. Balancing poses* to maintain physical and mental equilibrium: Pose of a Tree; Eagle Pose; Angular Pose. *Bending, stretching and breath-*

ing cycle, to benefit whole body: Greeting to the Rising Sun.
Relaxing Poses: Savasana – Pose of Complete Rest; *Advasana*;
Pose of a Child; Pose of a Hare; Modified Fish Pose.

So far we have only briefly mentioned one of the most vital
practices of yoga. The teaching concerning *prana* and the
method of yoga breathing must be thoroughly understood
from the very beginning. They are always explained at the
first lesson for they are the basis on which the whole system
is built. Without them physical exercise loses its full power
and becomes little more than gymnastics.

The word *hatha* comes from the Sanscrit: *ha*, the sun,
signifying the breath flowing through the right nostril, and
tha, the moon, symbolic of the breath through the left
nostril. *Hatha* yoga thus means Union of the Sun and Moon
breaths, and when this is achieved the mind is completely
stilled; it enters the state of higher consciousness called
samadhi, in which yoga is attained and man's spirit is united
with God.

Union of the two breaths also gives the yogi complete
control over *prana*, the primal energy.

Prana is a Sanscrit word meaning Vital Energy, Life Force,
Cosmic Energy; it is the power that keeps the world turning,
that keeps us alive. It exists in the sea, in the earth, above all
in the air, and without it we would soon perish.

'As fire, *Prana* burns; as the sun he shines; as cloud he
rains; as Indra he rules the gods; as wind, he blows, as the
moon he nourishes all. He is that which is visible, also that
which is invisible. He is immortal life.'

That is how *prana* is described in the Upanishads.

To a certain extent we take *prana* into the system through
different parts of the body ... the pores, the tips of the
fingers ... but mainly through the lungs in breathing. When
breathing is shallow and inadequate, less *prana* is absorbed;
when it is a full complete breath, using the whole of the
lungs, the maximum *prana* is inhaled. The more inhaled, the
greater the vitality, the better the health, the more vigorous
the outlook; the longer we remain youthful.

Prana holds the body together. When we can no longer
take it in, the body dies and soon afterwards decomposes.

25

Prana is inhaled but NOT exhaled. It remains in the system, accumulating and building up reserves of energy. If our supplies of *prana* are low we become weak, tired and old before our time.

This *pranic* theory must be accepted without reservation by all serious students, for it is a fundamental part of yoga philosophy. The higher forms of training are all devoted to the control of breath or so-called *pranayama* techniques; it is believed that as an adept acquires this control of breath, and thus control of the Life Force, he could even acquire control over life itself.

Anyone who retains reservations about *prana*'s presence in the air would do well to remember that fifty-odd years ago any talk of Vitamin D in sunlight or Vitamin C in orange juice would have been considered insane.

This intake, retention and accumulation of *prana*, which is the great focus of *Hatha* yoga training, is achieved through various breathing exercises and techniques. These are numerous and all designed to send vital energy to the solar plexus, the seat of energy in the human body, or to any other desired part. Establishing deep and rhythmical breathing, the student forms a mental image of the Life Force being stored in the solar plexus or directed through the nervous channels to vital organs or nerve centres. This concentration on the solar plexus, performed while breath is retained, is followed right through most of the cycles of breathing exercises.

The three main kinds of cycles are Recharging Breaths for increasing energy through inhaling *prana*; Purifying Breaths, for cleansing the bloodstream and emptying out stale air from the lungs; and Pacifying Breaths, for relaxing the nerves, and calming the mind and emotions. There are also breathing techniques for cooling or warming the body, for healing, for use in mental training and meditation. Some of these are only for advanced students but there are plenty of simple and harmless exercises suitable for beginners.

For ordinary students, the main benefits and reasons for correct breathing are:

1. To relax tension.
2. To overcome fatigue and to increase and replenish energy.
3. To calm the mind, nerves and emotions, and to improve sleep.
4. To purify the blood by supplying more oxygen for the body cells.
5. To improve memory, concentration and all mental processes.
   (Deep breathing is an essential preliminary to meditation.)

Correct breathing can also control the weight through its effect on the metabolic processes. It brings clear skin, bright eyes and greater physical magnetism.

First, the correct way to breathe must be learnt. It is not difficult, only perhaps a little unfamiliar at first.

So-called 'normal' breathing is an incorrect and shallow form of respiration which uses only the top part of the lungs. It does not take in enough fresh air or exhale enough stale air; it leaves a permanent reservoir of impure air in the lungs which slowly poisons the system, causing headaches, insomnia, fatigue, lack of energy, mental slowness. The body becomes like a room that is never ventilated.

The yoga breath is a complete breath which uses the maximum lung capacity, taking in the maximum of fresh air and exhaling the maximum of stale air. It is described as a diaphragm breath and is often taught by physiotherapists in asthma cases, and by singing or elocution teachers. It is used in public speaking and wherever breath control is needed.

Always breathe in and out through the nose unless you are told otherwise.

Stand straight, or lie on your back, and put your hands lightly on your waistline with fingertips just touching (Fig. 1A).

Breathe in through the nose and at the same time let the abdomen come forward, like a frog inflating itself when it breathes. If you are practising properly your fingertips should move apart as the abdomen swells out (Fig. 1B).

Breathe out, through the nose, drawing in the stomach so the fingertips come together again.

Remember that the abdomen comes *out* as you breathe *in*, and goes *in* as you breathe *out*.

Practise these first movements till they are quite familiar; then try the full breath.

With fingertips on the waistline, inhale, with abdomen coming forward. As you continue to breathe in, expand your lower ribs, then the middle ribs, then the upper ribs and top of the chest. Expand, *not* pull up. When you have taken in all the air you want, breathe out, drawing in the abdomen as before.

Read this carefully a couple of times before you start to practise. It may sound complicated but once you start you will find that you are automatically breathing in one smooth continuous movement. It is our natural method of respiration. If you watch an animal or a young baby lying down you will see that when they breathe they move the whole abdomen, not just the top of the chest.

The movement of the abdomen is very important. As it comes forward the diaphragm is flattened and the bottom of the lungs begin to fill with air. As you continue inhaling the lungs gradually fill right up. When you draw in the stomach to exhale, the diaphragm returns to its normal position and the lungs empty out all the stale air.

The best way to practise this breathing is lying on your back – perhaps in bed at night when you can concentrate quietly – or in the Pose of a Frog, (page 86), sitting back on the heels, with toes together, knees wide apart and palms together over the head.

The yoga breathing rate is slower than usual – about 6 units or heartbeats to breathe in and 6 to breathe out. This peaceful slow rhythm not only gives more time for the oxygen and *prana* to work in the body, but also relaxes tension and quietens the whole system.

Breathing is a very complex subject but in the beginning you need only learn how it is done. You must be quite familiar with it so you can do it automatically while you are practising your *asanas*, otherwise you will become very confused. In Chapters Four and Five you will find breathing cycles which you can do at home.

Remember that by taking in more air you are also taking

in more oxygen and *prana*. A simple demonstration of *prana*'s immediate effect is to get out of a closed car or train up in the mountains and take a deep breath. You at once notice a difference and begin to feel full of energy. This is because the air is charged with unpolluted *prana*; but even in the cities we could learn to increase our supply by proper breathing.

Remember, too, that mental concentration is essential, as one of the three powers needed for success in yoga: power of the breath, power of the mind and power of bodily position (*asana*).

Yoga breathing should not only be confined to exercises; it can become a valuable aid in everyday life. We all know the connection between the emotions and breath; in anger, fear, excitement the heart beats more quickly, the breathing accelerates; in peaceful or happy situations the breath comes more slowly.

Reversing this natural phenomenon, yoga consciously calms the mind by slowing the breath rate. Under the quieter rhythmical respiration the nerves relax, angry or hurtful words remain unspoken, tranquillity replaces hatred or despair. The most everyday situations and ordeals – a dreaded dental appointment, an important interview, a public appearance – could all be made less harassing by steadying the nerves through breath control. It could even reduce pain when combined with conscious relaxation of muscles and nerves, and mental concentration on a point outside yourself.

The following incident gives some idea of the power and practical use of yoga breathing.

One weekend I received a telephone call, in the country, from a woman in great distress. She was a distinguished musician and was to give a recital next day on television before thousands of viewers. She had been working too hard and had suddenly broken down; she had completely lost her nerve, her mind was a blank and she could not remember a note. She was desperate. Though I was a stranger she had read one of our yoga books and rung my house in Sydney. When she heard I was out of town she had begged for my country number and implored me to help her. Since I could not go to town that day I suggested she come to me. She drove the sixty-odd miles and arrived in a state of nervous collapse.

We went to a secluded part of the garden and after an hour or more of relaxing, deep breathing and various *asanas* she became calmer. When she had fully learnt the yoga breath and how to use it she went home, promising not to look at her work, to go straight to bed and next morning to practise deep breathing as soon as she woke. She was to do it on the drive home from the country and on the way to her recital next day, also while waiting to perform and while she played.

Thanks to this breath control she survived her ordeal successfully and calmly. She later described it as having 'saved her life'.

In the West, the power of the breath is still far from fully appreciated, though medical scientists are aware of its healing properties. In some countries breathing clinics have been established where the only treatment is rest and breathing exercises. It is known, too, that breathing can change the chemical composition of the blood and bring about certain states of mind, and researchers are now investigating the ancient yoga belief that due to incorrect respiration four-fifths of the human brain is never developed. Only one-fifth is used by most of us; the rest lies dormant, starved of nourishment for the cells, except in those yogis who through knowledge of breath control can awaken it and bring it to full power.

The *siddhis* or special powers of advanced yogis include levitation, the power to rise in the air. Western students who cannot accept tales of ancient sages travelling through space may be interested in the case of Nijinsky, the great Russian dancer, who was famous for his extraordinary power of elevation. Hundreds of people have described him as leaping into the air and seeming to stay there, coming down *slowly*. He said he had learnt how to do it from his father, also a dancer, and that it was done *through the breath*.

Chapter Three

PRACTISING AT HOME

Teachers are often asked what is the minimum time for practice and what it should include (see suggested practice lists on pp. 152-8). The answer is that there is really no short cut in yoga; yet everyone cannot spend long hours in practice. There are many students who genuinely want to make progress but whose time is literally not their own. In such cases, a little is better than nothing, so long as it is done in a peaceful relaxed mood. It is not much good sacrificing something else for practice if you are worried or harassed about it.

The exercises and *asanas* in the next chapter have been arranged in the form of a lesson, and when performed with time between for relaxing should take about an hour. This full practice is recommended for those who have reasonable freedom, preferably to be done at the same time every day, so that the body will come to expect it regularly and the effects will be stronger.

The most suitable hour is the one most convenient, so long as it is not less than three hours after a meal. Midday is a good time; by then you have digested breakfast, your muscles have been warmed up and afterwards you can eat lunch in a relaxed mood and be fresh for the afternoon and evening.

If your job makes this impossible or if you are so tied that your freedom is minimal, practise first thing in the morning. This is always the best time for breathing exercises and stomach contractions, and though you may be stiff after the night and have difficulty doing certain *asanas*, a warm shower will help to loosen you up.

If a whole hour all at once is impossible, split the practice and do breathing and stomach contractions when you get up, and half an hour of *asanas* at midday, if you are at home. If you go to work and live alone – that is, if you don't have to cook family meals and get children off to school – you could do a few minutes stretching and breathing when you first get out of bed, practise stomach contractions under the shower or in the bathroom, and when you come home after work lie down in *Savasana* for a few minutes, then do some *asanas* before dinner. If you are too tired and hungry for yoga before eating you will have to wait till just before bedtime. In this case, include relaxing and pacifying breaths so you don't get into bed overstimulated and unable to sleep.

Serious students who work in jobs sometimes practise in their lunch-hour, if they can find a suitable place. But yoga should never be hurried. In traditional practice, *asanas* are held for far longer periods than is possible in a Western class where time is limited, so the next best thing is to do them as slowly as possible, holding them as long as you can.

Choose a quiet spot where you will not be disturbed, spread your mat or rug and lie down on your back. The lesson starts with an exercise in relaxation known as *Savasana*, Pose of Complete Rest, or Corpse Pose. It is done on the floor because that is the best place to relax.

You should not practise while body and mind retain tension. If it is not first discharged, exertion will build it up into over-stimulation. This could be compared to going to bed over-tired and over-excited and lying awake, unable to sleep because of taut nerves and over-active brain.

In a group or class this preliminary relaxation has an additional purpose. Pupils arriving for a lesson are usually in different states of mind: cheerful, depressed, tense, worried, harassed, out of breath from hurrying, with minds full of the day's events. *Savasana* brings them all down to the same level of peace and tranquillity and prepares them for practice.

Learning to relax is one of the most difficult of all exercises, but when mastered it gives absolute refreshment. Starting with the simple relief of just lying down, one proceeds to deeper and more complete release of tension until finally, one day, one 'comes to' and realises that one has just not been there at all, in a sense; not asleep but far away in a tranquil and beautiful place. One returns as from an absence, full of peace and well-being.

This feeling will not come until all nervous energy has been withdrawn and the mind detached from its usual preoccupations. We all have this power of withdrawal, although we may not cultivate it consciously. It is more often used unconsciously, as when we become absent-minded or so sunk in thought that we do not hear when spoken to, and pass friends in the street without seeing them.

You may practise this Pose of Complete Rest for as long and as often as you like, at different times during the day. It can do nothing but good.

If you are harassed when you start your practice and find it hard to let yourself go, take a deep breath, tensing all your muscles, then exhale and relax them. Do this several times.

The secret of relaxing is yoga breathing.

Even after tension is discharged you should not start practice with 'cold' muscles. When you have finished *Savasana*, warm them up, as a dancer does, with preliminary exercises.

Certain movements and poses (marked in the text with an asterisk★) must be included every time, whether in class or at home. Yoga is a combination of bodily training and tonic therapy which should be repeated regularly if it is to have its effect. *Asanas* to tone up glands, breathing cycles to mantain energy, techniques for purification and movements to keep spine and joints supple cannot do their work if they are performed only at long intervals.

After warming up, at least five minutes should be spent on breathing exercises for recharging the body with energy, purifying the bloodstream and pacifying the nerves. You could vary the cycles, but should always include one of each group.

Breathing cycles should be followed by selected exercises or some of the series of Slow Movements for developing and moulding various parts of the body.

After the exercises, lie down, slow your breathing and relax in one of the relaxing poses given in the text. Never go on from one exertion to the next without relaxing in between. It is this alternating stimulation and pacification throughout the lesson that gives the refreshment.

After a few minutes of slow peaceful breathing you are ready to start the *asanas*. They must be done slowly, with full concentration.

Beginners complain that they find it hard to concentrate, which is perfectly natural since few people have ever consciously tried to develop this faculty. Improving it is a most important part of yoga training, but it will not happen overnight. You must persevere, helping yourself with deep breathing, which is the key to controlling the mind.

Some of the positions could be varied on different days: for instance you could start with balancing poses one day and the next with *Surya Namaskar* or Greeting to the Rising Sun, a combined breathing, bending and stretching cycle.

If some of the balancing poses seem difficult at first, you should remember that they are designed to cultivate both physical and mental equilibrium and that 50% of your effort should be in mental concentration. Focus your eyes on an unmoving spot and try to keep your whole attention upon it while maintaining deep and calm breathing. In practising balancing poses never make sudden or jerky movements or watch moving objects.

After further short relaxation comes the group known as Inverted Poses. These are extremely important and must always be included. Relax between each one – there are four – and at the end of the cycle.

Asanas which bend the spine in the opposite way to the Inverted Poses are usually practised next; then after further relaxation, the student sits in one of the cross-legged poses for breathing techniques, exercises for eyes, head, neck, facial muscles. Stomach contractions and mental exercises may also be done in sitting position. This stage of the lesson forms a break between the Inverted Poses and the Stretching Cycle which follows.

In sitting positions, whether in a cross-legged pose or as preliminary to a stretching *asana*, the back and head must always be held in one straight line. This is very important, not only for the health of the spine and for general posture but also to facilitate correct movements.

The next set of *asanas* which twist and stretch the spine forward, sideways and backward, are all designed to keep it supple and healthy, to stimulate circulation to the roots of the spinal nerves, to firm up muscles and limber up the joints.

The last part of the hour includes various *asanas*, such as the Raised Poses, followed by *Savasana*. Relaxing is always easier at the end than at the beginning of practice.

The Headstand and its variations are done after *Savasana*, when the body has been brought back to a tranquil state.

During this hour, if you have followed this sequence, you will have exercised every part of the body.

Before you start to practise, select the *asanas* and exercises you need, learn them as well as you can, then work them into the lesson. Be sure to keep the balance between stimulation and pacification. If there is too much exertion and not enough relaxing you will be tired or over-stimulated; if there is not enough exercise the system will not be properly toned up.

With each *asana* in this book you will find a description of its purpose, its benefits, and, possibly, *Cautions and Prohibitions*. Once more it must be repeated that the latter must be carefully observed, particularly in cases of high blood-pressure, certain heart conditions, ulcers, spinal troubles and pregnancy. And even if the warnings do not apply to you, you must use commonsense and knowledge of your own body in selecting and practising the poses.

If you are out of training, do not worry about being stiff next day. If you practise correctly at a slow tempo, with plenty of relaxation, your only after-effects will be an increased sense of well-being . . .

Keep an open mind and always be ready to learn. Read as much as you can about yoga and remember that the secret of successful practice lies in three powers: power of the breath, power of bodily position (*asana*) and power of the mind (concentration).

Chapter Four

HATHA YOGA IN THE FORM OF A LESSON

★*SAVASANA*

The exercise is in four stages.

1. Lying on your back, shut your eyes and try to forget whatever may have been worrying or disturbing you during the day. Forget everything but the thought of relaxing. The arms should be by the sides, legs together but not stiff. Do not cross the ankles or bend the elbows; do not put your hands under your neck. Bending the limbs creates muscular tension, which is what you are trying to discharge.

   Starting from the toes, work up through the body, relaxing every group of muscles in turn: feet, ankles, calves, knees, thighs.

   Relax the stomach muscles, the muscles in the waist and small of the back.

   Relax the chest and shoulders, arms, hands and fingers.

   Relax the neck muscles.

   Let the lower jaw sag.

   Let the tongue go limp.

   Let your eyes turn back under the lids.

   Smooth out your forehead. Wipe out any frowning or tension between the eyebrows.

   There should not be a muscle tensed anywhere. Slowly and carefully check through the body to see that you have not missed any part. You could be still unconsciously clenching your fists, or the jaw might be set; there could be a harassed expression on your face or a tightness in the stomach muscles or small of the back – habits developed over long years of tension.

   If you find such areas, persuade the muscles to let go. It is no good ordering them to relax; the reaction will be increased tension. People who try too hard often defeat their object; a more relaxed approach will have greater success.

The breath should be slow and rhythmical, the full yoga breath with the abdomen coming forward with inhalation and going back with exhalation. This peaceful rhythmical breathing is your control, the key to your relaxing. By slowing the breath you are slowing the heart and quietening the whole system. You are also taking in *prana*, but not exhaling it. As you breathe out the stale air, focus your mind on the thought of the *prana* being sent all through your body, as food for the nerves, accumulating in the solar plexus, the seat of energy, building up a reserve.

2. *Withdrawal of Nervous Energy.* Having persuaded your muscles to soften and relax until you feel you have no bones at all, begin the release of your inner tension. This is much more difficult than relaxing the muscles and once more you must work gently and patiently, using a mild form of self-hypnosis.

   You cannot command your nerves to relax; it is better to try to create soothing images and thoughts in your mind, like the tide going out . . . water slowly ebbing away from the shore . . . and identify yourself with them, with the slow sense of withdrawal.

   Let the tension drain away from your nerves. Let go; there is no need to hold on. Let yourself drift. Let yourself sink, as one sometimes does just before falling asleep. Feel yourself sinking down, down into the darkness, even down through the floor. There is no need to move, to do anything.

   All messages from the brain have ceased; the central intelligence system has closed down; you don't care about anything; you can't be bothered, you're too indolent to think.

   As the inner tension, the stress and strain disperse there comes an extraordinary sensation of lightness, almost of being disembodied. The body is so tranquil, so completely at rest you are no longer conscious of it; only of the slow steady rhythm of breathing.

3. The third stage is called *Small Exit from the Physical Body.** In this you try to detach yourself mentally and send your

---

*The Great Exit from the Physical Body comes with death.

37

mind far away, escaping from your everyday life and present surroundings to some peaceful and beautiful place which you create in your imagination. It could perhaps be somewhere you know and love, a garden, a beach, the banks of a river, a mountain or country scene, but whatever it is, be really *there* more than here. Leave your body lying on the floor and let the real You escape, miles away to this tranquil *ashram* or retreat where nothing can hurt or worry you. Make it a true escape, leaving all your problems and responsibilities behind, so that you come back mentally refreshed.

4. The last stage is the hardest of all, when you must switch off all thoughts or mental pictures and try to keep the mind empty. This may seem impossible for a beginner; the minute one starts to try, every thought imaginable crowds into the head and one cannot control them. Yet countless people have mastered this important stage of *Savasana* by quiet perseverence.

Your greatest help is the breathing rate, the slow and rhythmical inhaling-exhaling which you have been practising all the time. Make it as slow as is comfortable – the slower the more powerful – and roll your eyes back under the lids, a traditional aid to emptying the mind.

Finally, open your eyes, stretch your arms, yawn, as though getting up in the morning, and stand up.

The duration of the four different stages depends on yourself – the longer the better – but spend at least two minutes on each.

★*LIMBERING UP*

PURPOSE: To warm up the muscles and prepare the body for further exercise; to stimulate the flow of arterial blood to the spine and the roots of the spinal nerves; to keep the spine supple.

1. Standing straight, with arms hanging loosely by the sides, slowly move both shoulders up and back, like a slow shrug; bring them down, forward, up and back again; down, forward, up and back in a continuous circular motion. You should feel the movement in the

small of the back as well as the shoulder area and a pleasant tingling sensation along the spine. *Repeat the movement four times.*

2. Reverse the movement. Bring the shoulders forward as though hunching them, then down, back, up; forward, down, back, up; etc, making sure you feel the movement in the spine. *Repeat four times.*

3. Rotate each shoulder separately but simultaneously. [Fig. 3 A to F] Bring the RIGHT shoulder up, in the slow shrugging movement, then back, down, forward, up and back again. AT THE SAME TIME, bring the LEFT shoulder down, forward, back, up and forward. The movement of the shoulders is alternating but simultaneous, designed to rotate the bones of the spine in their sockets. As the shoulders make their circular movements the vertebrae are slightly and gently twisted from side to side.

 The mind should be fully concentrated on the benefits of the cycle on the spine, which is being exercised through backward, forward and twisting movements, and a mental image formed in the Mind's Eye of the vertebrae rotating as the shoulders move. *Practise eight times; four times for each shoulder.*

Beginners often tend to put too much emphasis on moving the arms, as distinct from the shoulders. They must remember that the spine is the real focus of the exercise. The arms should hang loosely, not be consciously manipulated; they just go along with the shoulders as they are moved.

1. Now, standing with feet apart, let your body fall forward from the waist, as limply as possible. Let the arms and head flop like a rag doll.

 Come up and *repeat several times.* This relaxes tension as well as firming and slimming the waistline.

2. Let your body fall from the waist over to the right; then forward, across and up on the left side.

 Let it fall to the left, forward, across and up on the right.

 Practise four times, twice on each side.

3. Fall to the right, forward and across; up to the left and back and across to the right again; forward, across to

the left, up, back and across to the right, a continuous rolling movement, feeling it in the spine and small of the back.

Come up, bring your feet together, and with eyes either closed or focused on the tip of the nose, practise the following Pacifying Cycle for quietening the heart.

★NINE PACIFYING BREATHS

PURPOSE: To calm the mind and nerves in a very short time. Recommended for practice before bed, by an open window, if troubled with insomnia.

All inhalation and exhalation is through the nose.

1. *Practise four times.* Inhale and raise the arms forward and up, crossing them in front of the face, separating them and bringing them down at the sides in a circular movement, exhaling as they come down.
2. *Practise three times.* Inhale, bringing the arms up from the sides till the finger-tips touch above the head. Exhale and slowly lower them to the sides.
3. *Practise twice.* Inhale, raising the arms slowly forward and up over the head, keeping them parallel. Exhale and lower them.

In all these movements, inhalation takes place while the arms are raised, exhalation while they are lowered. The rhythm of breathing is extremely slow, not less than six counts for incoming, six for outgoing breath. The mind should be concentrated on peace . . . tranquillity.

Now start to increase your energy through Recharging exercises.

★VIGOROUS RECHARGING CYCLE
Inhale through the nose, exhale through the mouth.

1. Inhale deeply, lock the breath in the chest. Stretch the arms forward, clench the fists and bring them back against the chest, shaking the entire body. (Shaking the body while breath is retained speeds up and intensifies purification). Exhale.

Concentrate on the thought that you are exhaling only stale air, retaining the *prana* in your solar plexus.

2. Inhale. Stretch the arms forward and, with breath locked in the chest, swing them apart to the sides at shoulder height, then together again. *Repeat twice*, then drop the arms to the sides while exhaling through the mouth.
3. Inhale, swinging the arms up and then down, up again, down again, slightly arching the back. Exhale.
4. Inhale deeply, lock the breath and vigorously swing the arms, like windmills, twice backwards, twice forward. Exhale.
5. Inhale. Bend the body, from the waist, to the left, then to the right. As you bend swing the arms up to cross over the head; then down; then up again as you bend to the other side. Exhale.

Remember all through the cycle to concentrate on the thought of *prana* being inhaled and stored in the body, and stale air being exhaled.

Follow this cycle with the HA Breath or Cleansing Breath.

★*HA BREATH*
   With feet apart, inhale, raising the arms up from the sides till they are stretched over the head.
   When the lungs are full, exhale vigorously, throwing the upper part of the body forward, letting head and arms hang down as though to touch the toes.
   This strong exhalation is made with the sound HA, as you drive all the stale air out of the lungs.

   Repeat three times.

PRELIMINARY EXERCISES
The following selection is to be varied with other exercises taken from Chapter Five. Those marked † are from the cycle, *Magic of Slow Movements* (see page 82).

For legs and feet

To strengthen insteps, toe and foot muscles, flex hip and knee joints, limber up the ankles, firm the calves and thighs and improve circulation.

1. Standing with feet together, come up on the toes, then down; up – down; up – down, several times, stretching the insteps and feeling it in toe and foot muscles.

2. With feet apart and flat on the floor, bring the knees together, then apart; together –apart; together –apart, *six or seven times*, flexing knee joints and feeling it in the ankles, calves and thighs.

3. With hands on thighs, practise a half-squatting movement: down –up; down –up; down –up, *six or seven times*, flexing knee-joints and feeling it in calves and thighs.

4. Full squatting movement. With hands on hips, rise up on the toes, then squat right down on the heels. Come up and repeat, up –down –up; up –down –up, till pleasantly tired, feeling tension in the thighs and calf muscles, flexing hips, knees and ankles.

For the chest and waist

†1. Raise the arms and grasp an imaginary rope, pulling down on it, tensing the muscles at the side of the chest near the armpits. Relax and *repeat three times more*.

†2. Bring the arms up from the sides and then slowly down in front of the body, as though pressing against the air, tensing the chest muscles. *Practise four times*.

†3. Standing straight with arms at the sides. Imagine you have a very heavy weight or an iron dumbell in each hand. Bend to the right and slowly raise this heavy weight up till it is under the left arm-pit. Relax and lower the arm.

   Bend to the left and slowly pull the right hand up into the armpit.

   Relax. It is essential to really believe you have a weight to lift, otherwise the muscles will not tense properly. Continue bending and lifting, right, then left arm, *four times each side*.

For stomach, waistline and hips.

1. Lie on your back with hands clasped under your neck. Keeping the legs straight and together, slowly raise and lower them: up–down; up–down; up–down, *five times* without touching the ground in between. Relax.
2. Lying on the back with hands in the same position. Draw the right knee up towards the body, then stretch the leg out and draw up the left. Stretch the left out and draw up the right; stretch out the right and draw up the left. Continue this drawing-up and stretching-out with alternate legs until pleasantly tired. Do not bring the legs to the ground until finished.
3. On the back, with hands behind the neck, raise and lower right and left legs alternately in a scissors movement, without touching the ground. Continue until pleasantly tired.

    The reason for not bringing the legs down to the ground between movements is to make the stomach muscles do the work of supporting them.

Follow the preliminary exercises with a few quiet breaths, inhaling and exhaling through the nose.

1. Inhale, raising the arms over the head and placing the palms together. Exhale, lowering them.
2. Inhale, raising the arms and placing palms together before the chest. Exhale, lowering them.
3. Inhale, raising the arms above the head. Place palms together and bring them down in front of the chest. Exhale, and lower to the sides.

After this, practise a Balancing Pose, such as Pose of an Eagle.

POSE OF AN EAGLE (Fig. 4)
Remember that Balancing Poses are 50% physical, 50% mental concentration.
PURPOSE: To develop physical balance and inner tranquillity. Strengthens the ankles and legs; stimulates the sex glands in the lower abdomen by putting pressure on them. (Although the Eagle Pose is recommended as a remedy for infertility it

is also, when accompanied by appropriate mental techniques, practised as a sublimation exercise by celibate yogis.)

Stand with legs together.

Slightly bend the right leg.

Bring the left leg round it from the front, intertwining the legs with the left foot hooked behind the right calf (as though sitting on a high stool with legs twined).

Bend forward slightly and intertwine the arms, as if repeating the position of the legs. The elbow of the lower arm rests on the left thigh. The chin is pressed to the back of the upper hand.

The eyes are focused on the tip of the nose.

Hold the pose, deeply and rhythmically inhaling and exhaling.

Then change sides and repeat, standing on the left leg, with the right twined round.

Inhale, raising the arms over the head till the fingers touch.

Exhale, lowering them.

Repeat, then practise Stomach Contractions.

★UDDIYANA

CAUTION. Strictly forbidden in cases of stomach or duodenal ulcers, prolapse, and during menstruation and pregnancy. Only to be practised in normal health and on an empty stomach. Never to be done for at least three hours after a meal, particularly after eating fish.

PURPOSE: Essential to correct constipation and improve digestive system. Also firms and slims the stomach. Helps to regulate menstruation, when practised *between* periods. Gives deep internal massage. An extremely important *asana* which should be always included in practice, either in sitting or standing position. For best effect should be done daily, before breakfast and before opening the bowels.

Standing position
1.   Stand with feet about 18 in. apart.

  Place the palms flat on the thighs, high up with fingers pointing inwards.

Inhale.

Completely exhale, leaning forward and resting the weight on the hands. At the same time slightly bend the knees and arch the back, protruding the behind. It is not an elegant stance, but it gives maximum control.

Contract the abdominal muscles, pulling the stomach in and back, as far as you can towards the spine. There should be a deep cave under the ribs.

The chin is pressed to the chest.

Hold the contraction for a few seconds, then relax. *Repeat*.

2. Having drawn in the stomach, relax briefly and let it out, then quickly draw it in again. Repeat this in-out-in-out movement to the best of your ability. The contracting and relaxing of muscles eventually gives a flapping movement of the abdomen which becomes quicker and smoother with practice.

No one can actually teach you this *asana*, even by personal demonstration; it has to be attempted and practised continually, faithfully following directions until one day the muscles suddenly obey you. Read also the suggestions for practising *Nauli*.

★*NAULI*

CAUTION: As for *Uddiyana*.

PURPOSE: As for *Uddiyana*, although being a more advanced technique it has stronger and more powerful effects on digestive and eliminative systems.

Having mastered drawing-in the stomach for *Uddiyana*, the abdominal recti muscles are isolated by contraction, forming a column up the middle of the abdomen (see illustration). Then the muscles on the right side are contracted. Then the central muscles. Then muscles on the left side. Then central muscles . . . and so on . . . left, centre, right, centre, left . . .

When actually practised there is a continuous wave-like rolling movement from left to right across the abdomen and back.

PRACTICE NOTE: This is a very difficult exercise for most people and requires complete re-education of the abdominal muscles, but it is so important it should be mastered.

When trying to contract the central muscles in *Nauli*, stand in the same position as for *Uddiyana*, with feet about 18 in. apart and palms on the thighs, with fingers facing inwards.

Inhale, completely exhale and lean forward, taking the weight on the hands. At the same time make a downward thrusting movement at the pit of the stomach. This isolates the muscles at their base and forms them into a column. It gives you a better control. Relax them and try to isolate the muscles at the side.

The power of the mind is extremely important in both *Uddiyana* and *Nauli*, even to the point of self-hypnosis. Some authorities recommend practising in front of a mirror, others believe in the power of the Mind's Eye. This could be e most successful method.

To learn this way, establish position, completely exhale, shut your eyes and visualise the movement you are trying to learn, as if watching someone else doing it. Then imagine that you are also doing the movements, as though copying an imaginary demonstrator.

Keep trying, with the mind focused on this mental image, and suddenly, one day, if you persevere, you will find that your body is automatically responding: it begins to obey you and perform the correct movements.

Trying too hard, consciously, could have the opposite effect; the muscles stiffen up and resist your commands. When hypnotised, relaxed and persuaded, they become docile and obedient.

After the Stomach Contractions – you may do either or both *Uddiyana* and *Nauli* – lie down and relax. Slow down your breathing, resting the fingertips on the solar plexus and concentrating on the thought of *prana* being taken into the system but not breathed out again. The finger-tips on the solar plexus are closing the circuit of energy in the body; you are, as it were, tapping yourself to your own source of vitality.

After a few minutes of this combined relaxing and re-charging, come up into the Shoulderstand.

★SHOULDERSTAND OR CANDLE POSITION

CAUTION: If you have spinal disc weakness, be careful with the second part of this *asana*, when bringing the legs down over the head. Avoid jerking or sudden movements. If there is any weakness or deterioration of vertebrae in the back of the neck, be very careful about putting pressure on that area. If painful, see a doctor and ask if you should practise this pose.

PURPOSE: By sending extra arterial blood to the thyroid and parathyfoid glands and thus toning-up and regulating them, this pose benefits the entire endocrinal system and conse-quently the whole body. It delays ageing, increases vitality, ontrols the weight, improves the metabolic processes. It also helps to resist the downward pull of central gravity, keeps the spine supple, prevents and even cures varicose veins. It helps women going through the menopause by reducing the dis-comfort of hot flushes and mental depression. It is essential in any weight-reducing programme.

Lie on your back with the legs together and arms by the sides. Slowly lift the legs, then the body, as high as you can into a vertical position. (Eventually, with practice, legs and back should make one straight line.)

Prop yourself up with your hands, placing them against your back in the area of the shoulderblades. Keep the elbows close to the sides.

Press the chin firmly to the chest.

Make yourself as comfortable as possible in the pose, shut your eyes and establish deep and rhythmical breathing (Fig. 7A).

The mind should be concentrated on the thought that this is a powerful medium for increasing vigour and vitality, a key pose in rejuvenation and benefiting the whole system. Constructive thinking is essential.

The deep respiration is also essential. To do its work, the arterial blood sent to the thyroid must be oxygenated; it is useless to bring unpurified blood to the glands.

Hold the pose for as long as you comfortably can.

Slowly lower the legs over the head till the toes touch the floor, if possible.

Bring the arms back to the floor and briefly rest the toes on the floor (this is called the Plough Pose, Fig. 7B).

Inhale and exhale, concentrating the mind on the spinal column and on the thought that the roots of the spinal nerves are being toned-up and supplied with rich arterial blood.

Then begin to come back to starting point, slightly bending the knees and slowly lowering them till you are lying flat on the floor again.

Relax for a few minutes before attempting the next pose.

NEVER jump up immediately after holding any inverted poses. Lie quietly, allowing the blood circulation to return to normal.

Shoulderstand is one of the most important of all yoga *asanas*. Everyone should make an effort to master it, unless there is some physical prohibition; it should always be included in practice and, if possible, done every day. If at first you are not strong enough to hold it, support your legs against a wall or heavy table. (The inclining boards used as health and beauty aids were inspired by the inverted positions).

At first, maintain the pose only for a short time, no more than two minutes, but gradually increase it to five or even more. The longer it is held the more time the blood has to drain from the legs and body and travel to the thyroid glands, where it is stopped by the pressure of the chin.

★*HALF-SHOULDERSTAND*

CAUTION: *Strictly forbidden* in cases of high blood-pressure. Be careful if there is any spinal disc weakness.

PURPOSE: This is known as Anti-wrinkle Pose but for full effect it must be practised regularly at the same time every day for a considerable period. It nourishes the facial tissues by sending extra arterial blood to the face, feeds the teeth, gums, eyes and hair, also nerve centres and glands in the head. It exercises the spine and keeps it supple, discourages fat on stomach and waistline and prevents and corrects varicose veins.

Lying on the back, with arms by the sides, raise the legs and body as in the Shoulderstand.

Support yourself by holding the hips (instead of the back), with the body at an angle of 30° from the vertical. The legs should be completely vertical.

Do not press the chin to the chest; keep the head back so the blood can flow freely to the face. You should feel a warmth and fullness in the cheeks.

Close the eyes and relax the facial muscles (Fig. 8A).

Hold the pose as long as you comfortably can, deeply inhaling and exhaling. Concentrate on the image of yourself 'youthful and unchangeable'.

Then bring the legs down slowly over the head.

Bend the knees, take hold of your toes and pull the legs out straight and down, until the toes are resting on the floor, in the Plough Pose (Fig. 8B).

Retain the position, inhaling and exhaling, and concentrating on the spinal nerves being supplied with arterial blood, and on the spine being kept supple.

Let go the toes, slightly bend the legs and lower them slowly till you are lying flat, with the arms by the sides.

Relax completely before the next *asana*.

★ *POSE OF TRANQUILLITY or TRIANGULAR POSE*

CAUTION: Use care in second part (Choking Pose) if there is spinal disc weakness.

PURPOSE: Essential in cases of insomnia for its power in promoting better and more restful sleep. Soothes the whole nervous system, improves poor circulation and helps to cure cold feet. Exercises the spine, contributes to general suppleness and discourages fat on waist and abdomen. The Choking Pose puts pressure on the thyroid gland and keeps it healthy and regulated.

Lie on the floor with arms by the sides.

49

Stretch the arms above your head (along the floor), then slowly raise the legs until they form an angle of 45° with the floor.

Raise the arms and rest the knees on the palms of the hands.

Arms, body and legs form a triangle (Fig. 9A).

The arms must be kept straight; if the elbows are bent the balance will be lost. In most cases the hands should be in the region of the knee-caps but the position varies with individual proportions. You must find your own position of balance according to the lengths of your arms and legs. Experiment by moving the hands along the legs until you find the balance. You will know immediately when you have it because the pose will become comfortable and the balance quite steady.

If balance is not correct the *asana* cannot do its work of sending extra arterial blood to a nerve centre at the back of the head, which is vitally connected with our powers of sleeping.

When balance is established, hold the pose as long as comfortable (the longer the better), deeply inhaling and exhaling, with the mind concentrated on thoughts of peace.

Bring the legs down over the head, with the knees bent.

Split the legs apart so that one is on each side of the head.

Put your hands on the backs of the knees and press them against the floor, one on each side of the head, in the Choking Pose, with chin pressed against the chest. Keep the feet flat against the floor; don't dig in the toes (Fig. 9B).

After holding briefly, release the knees and slowly lower the legs and arms to the floor.

Relax completely before the next *asana*.

★*BALANCING SHOULDERSTAND*
CAUTION: Be careful in Choking Pose, if there is spinal disc weakness.

PURPOSE: This pose completely reverses the circulation, sending extra arterial blood to the pineal gland. It rests and refreshes the arms and legs by draining them of blood, relieves and prevents varicose veins, resists the pull of gravity and strengthens the spine and back muscles. The Choking Pose tones up the thyroid gland.

Balancing Shoulderstand is also known to yogis as the Pose of Higher Faculties because of its effect on the pineal gland, the seat of higher powers such as clairvoyance, telepathy, clairaudience, etc.

Lie on the back with the arms by the sides.
Stretch the arms above the head, along the floor.
Raise the legs, then the body, as high as possible, as in the Shoulderstand, but without the support of the hands.
Try to balance on the back of the neck and head and top of the shoulders. Raise the arms and hold them in line with the legs, *without* touching them.
Hold the pose as long as comfortable, inhaling and exhaling, with the mind concentrated on the extra blood that is going to the pineal gland at the back of the head and helping to keep it healthy and regulated (Fig. 10A).
Bring the legs slowly down over the head.
Split the knees apart, as in Triangular Pose.
Put the hands on the backs of the knees and press them against the floor in the Choking Pose, with chin pressed against the chest (Fig. 10B).
Release the knees.
Bring the arms and legs down slowly to the floor.

Completely relax.
Then come into the Modified Fish Pose and continue relaxing, with deep and peaceful breathing.

MODIFIED FISH POSE
(In the full Fish Pose the legs must be locked in the Lotus Position. This adaptation is easier for beginners).

PURPOSE: This is an excellent pose in which to practise yoga breathing, particularly for beginners. The position of the legs facilitates the free movement of the diaphragm, the position of the arms makes it impossible to draw up the shoulders as in shallow breathing. Combined with yoga respiration it is highly recommended as a relaxing pose. It also exercises and flexes hip joints, knees and shoulder-blades.

Lying on your back, cross your legs and draw them up under you, towards the body.

Cross the arms behind the head. The left palm should be under the right shoulder; the right palm should be under the left shoulder. The head rests on the crossed arms (Fig. 11A).

Shut your eyes and hold the pose, deeply and rhythmically inhaling and exhaling.

Alternatively, place the fingertips on the diaphragm as described on page 46 (Fig. 11B).

Then turn over and lie on your stomach, with arms by your sides and face turned to one side. Relax for a couple of minutes, then prepare to practise the Pose of a Cobra.

★POSE OF A COBRA

CAUTION: Not advisable in later stages of pregnancy, due to pressure on the abdomen.

PURPOSE: Strengthens the spine and keeps it supple; increases energy and vitality by toning up the adrenal glands in the small of the back, which are squeezed as the spine is arched; helps to correct menstrual troubles and complaints of the female reproductive system by regulating the ovaries through pressure on the lower abdomen; facilitates full yoga breathing; firms the chest, waist, stomach and thigh muscles.

In the variation B, the thyroid gland is also toned up when the chin is pressed in. This benefits the whole body, increases energy, delays ageing, reduces weight and favourably influences all other glands, including the sex glands.

A. Lying face down, with chin and feet resting on the floor, place your palms on the floor, level with your shoulders.

Inhale, and at the same time very slowly begin to lift the front part of the body, arching the spine, with the head back.

Push yourself up by pressing with your hands against the floor. The lower part of the body, from the waistline down, should be pressed to the floor. There should be a pleasant sensation of pressure in the small of the back.

Hold the pose and the breath as long as comfortable (Fig. 12A).

Start to come down, very slowly, exhaling at the same time.

Relax.

Repeat the movements, combined with inhaling, breath retention and exhalation.

Relax.

B. Repeat twice more in exactly the same way but with the chin pressed in to the chest, not held back (Fig. 12B).

These movements must be done very slowly, and the breath should be held as long as possible without discomfort. Retention of breath is a very important part of the *asana*.

After the Cobra Pose, relax briefly, lying on the stomach with arms by the sides and face turned to one side, practising slow breathing. Then begin the Locust Pose.

★*POSE OF A LOCUST*
CAUTION: Avoid in cases of high blood-pressure.

PURPOSE: Benefits the lungs and the whole respiratory system; exercises the diaphragm and lower abdominal muscles. Limbers up the spine, invigorates the body through action on the adrenal glands; reduces fat on stomach and waistline; rejuvenates through sending arterial blood to the face.

Lie face downwards on the floor with the arms very close to the body (beginners should put them under the sides and thighs).

Clench the fists and turn them so that the thumb is underneath, resting on the floor.

Turn your face to one side.

Inhale, and, trying to keep the face on the floor,

Raise both legs in a quick movement, keeping them close together. Hold the breath and position as long as you comfortably can.

Lower the legs slowly, while exhaling.

Repeat once more.

Relax.

Do not hold the legs up too long, since breath is being retained.

Rest briefly, on the stomach with arms by the sides, practising slow breathing, before going on to the Bow Pose.

POSE OF A BOW

CAUTION: Do not practise late in pregnancy, nor for six months after an abdominal operation.

PURPOSE: Limbers up the spine; stimulates the spinal nerves and invigorates the whole body through action on the adrenal glands. Also firms the thighs and buttocks, slims the abdomen and firms and develops the bust.

Lie on the floor, face downward, with arms by your sides.

Bend back your legs and grasp your ankles.

Inhale, and at the same time raise head and shoulders, pulling on the ankles so that the body forms an arc.

Hold the pose and the breath for a couple of seconds (Fig. 14A).

Come down and relax.

Repeat once more.

Relax.

If your spine is, anyway, supple and your body forms a

good arc, vary the pose by rocking back and forth, while holding the ankles, like a rocking-horse. This massages the abdominal organs and reduces fat on the stomach.

Spinal Massage is very pleasant after these back-bending *asanas*.

Turn over on your back.

Cross your legs and draw them up towards your stomach, and clasp your hands round them.

Close your eyes and gently rock from side to side, as though in a cradle, massaging the roots of the spinal nerves (Fig. 14B).

Then sit up with your legs crossed.

★*EASY POSE*. Fig. 15

CAUTION: Although it puts no heavy pressure on the legs, this pose should be used with discretion if there are bad varicose veins. In such cases it should only be held for short periods, or with intervals when legs can be stretched and circulation restored before resuming the pose.

PURPOSE: To keep the back strong and hip and knee joints flexible. With time and practice the hip joints will loosen up, enabling you to bring the knees lower towards the floor.

Sit on the floor with the back and neck *in one straight line*. This is important.

Cross your legs and rest your hands on the knees, with thumb and forefinger joined, or hold them in the lap, one on the other, with palms turned up.

This is the simplest sitting pose for beginners, and is used constantly in yoga for breathing cycles, for relaxing, for mental exercises, and for meditation.

When you have established a steady and comfortable position, spend a few minutes quietening the system with a cycle of Pacifying Breaths.

PACIFYING BREATH

Controlled breath has a strong pacifying effect on the mind and whole nervous system. The normal breathing rate is 15–20 breaths a minute; in pacifying breathing the rate is slowed to 5–6 breaths a minute. The rhythm is established either by counting the heart or pulse beats with a finger on the wrist, or by concentrating on the syllable OHM, using it as a unit of counting: 6 heartbeats or 6 OHMS for inhalation, 6 for exhalation.

After a short period of this slow breathing, which helps to prepare the mind, practise the following mental exercise for developing the powers of concentration and imagination.

CREATING A FLOWER

With breath and pose established, shut your eyes and for a few seconds see only darkness. Then begin to create the image of a simple flower, behind your closed lids, using your Mind's Eye, your visual imagination. Choose a flower before starting the exercise, so that you are not distracted by uncertainty, and at first choose something familiar.

You must see the flower clearly, its colour, form, texture, and hold the image while deeply inhaling and exhaling. As you improve in concentration it will be easier to hold it for longer periods, even to imagine the scent as you inhale.

This exercise could be practised lying on your back in *Savasana*, or in bed at night. It is soothing and relaxing to mind and nerves.

Vary the image of the flower, at other times, by creating a beautiful garden or landscape or any other imaginary scene. Continue the concentration, helped by your deep breathing, as long as you like. Then open your eyes.

Bend to the right and touch your right knee with your forehead. Bend to the left and touch your left knee with your forehead. Take hold of your toes and lean forward, touching your forehead to the floor.

Stretch your legs and move them to restore circulation, then cross them again for Head and Neck, and Eye exercises.

HEAD AND NECK EXERCISES
Perform the first five movements four times

1. Raise the head; lower it; up-down; up-down; up-down.
2. Turn the head from left to right; then from right to left.
3. Slant the head towards the right shoulder, then to the left shoulder.
4. Raise the head, then let it fall forward limply on the chest.
5. Push the chin out and draw it in again (anti-double chin movement).
6. Rotate the head in a half-circle, to the right. Let it drop forward, then rotate in a half-circle to the left.
7. Rotate the head in a complete circle, to the left, then to the right.
8. With hands clasped on the back of the neck, press the head down and forward, at the same time resisting with the neck. (This strengthens the muscles at the back of the neck and helps to prevent the condition called 'Dowager's Hump'). Repeat three times.

Then practise the Eye Exercises. If you wear glasses, take them off first.

EYE EXERCISES
Moving only the eyes and each time focusing on a specific point:

1. Eyes up, down; up, down; up, down; close.
2. Eyes up; straight ahead; down; straight ahead; up; straight ahead; down; straight ahead; up; straight ahead; down; straight ahead; close.
3. Eyes left; right; left; right; left; right; close.
4. Eyes left; straight ahead; right; straight ahead; left; straight ahead; right; straight ahead; left; straight ahead; close.
5. Look up in a diagonal direction; then down in diagon-

ally opposite direction; up, right corner; down, left corner; up, right corner; down, left corner; up, right corner; down, left corner; close.

6. The same movement but changing the direction: up to the left corner, down to the right, etc.

7. Slowly circle the eyes, right round to the left; then close.
Slowly circle, round to the right. Close.

Changing of focus:

8. Look at the tip of your nose, then at a point in the distance; nose; distance; nose; distance; nose; distance; close.

9. Look at the tip of your finger, held about a foot away, then in the distance; finger; distance; finger; distance; finger; distance; close.

10. Look steadily at a chosen object without blinking, staring without strain, trying to see it more clearly.

11. Massage the eyes by squeezing the lids tightly together, then blinking rapidly several times.

12. Palming – put the palms over the closed eyes to completely exclude the light.

Now stretch your legs, move them about to restore circulation and proceed with the Forward-stretching Cycle.

★ARCH GESTURE

CAUTION: Since these movements bring blood to the head they are not recommended in cases of high blood-pressure. Where there is a history of spinal disc weakness they should be done with great care, avoiding any sudden jerks. Avoid Variation (iv) if there are varicose veins.

PURPOSE: Keeps spine and joints supple; reduces fat on stomach and waistline; rejuvenates facial tissues by bringing blood to the head; massages the internal organs.
Start from sitting position.
Stretch the right leg forward, bend the left knee and put the sole of the left foot flat against the right thigh.

The bent and the stretched legs should be at right angles to each other. The hands should rest on the knees, thumbs and index fingers joined. Head and back should be in one straight line. (Fig. 17A.)

Inhale.

Exhale, and bend forward, bringing the head down to touch the right knee and at the same time reach the arms forward till the fingers rest on the toes of the right foot, if possible. (Fig. 17B.)

Hold briefly, then come up.

Repeat.

Change sides and, sitting with left leg stretched, right leg bent and right sole pressed against the left thigh, practise twice more.

Variations of Arch Gesture

(i) With left leg stretched forward and right bent at the knee and the right foot under the left thigh.

Inhale; exhale and come forward, head to knee, both hands to the left foot.

Come up; then repeat.

Change sides and practise twice with right leg stretched.

(ii) Sit with left leg stretched forward and right leg drawn up close to the body, knee bent, foot flat on the floor and both hands resting on the stretched knee (Fig. 17C).

Inhale, exhale and come down, pressing the head to the stretched knee and putting the hands on the left foot (Fig. 17D).

Come up and repeat.

Change sides and practise twice with right leg stretched.

(iii) With left leg stretched and right leg bent back so the calf lies beside and close to the body. Rest the left hand on the left knee. Hold the right ankle with the right hand.

Inhale, exhale and come forward, pressing the head to the knee.

The right hand remains on the ankle.

The left hand comes forward to touch the toes of the left foot.

Come up.

Repeat.

Change sides and practise twice with right leg stretched.

(iv) Sit with left leg stretched forward. Lift the right foot with your hands and place it up in the groin, in the Half-Lotus position. Do not force it; just do the best you can, without straining. It becomes easier with practice. Rest the hands on the knees.

Inhale, exhale and come forward, pressing the head to the left knee and bringing the arms forward so that the fingers of both hands touch the toes of the left foot.

Come up.

Repeat.

Change sides and practise twice with the right leg stretched.

As you come forward, pull in the stomach; this helps to flatten and firm it. Each time the position of the bent leg is changed a different part of the abdominal organs is massaged when you lean forward. If you have trouble in reaching the toes, take hold of your ankle and give yourself a *gentle* tug forward and down.

Never strain or force the muscles; keep practising so that they loosen up naturally. Be sure not to bend the stretched leg. Once you start to cheat in this way you may never master the pose properly, whereas if you persevere correctly you will find it gets easier as you go on.

Now cross your legs, take hold of your toes, inhale and exhale as you come forward, trying to touch the floor with the forehead, without rising up at the back.

POSE OF A STAR

CAUTION: Not for those with high blood-pressure. To be practised carefully when there is any history of spinal disc displacement or weakness. Avoid jerking or sudden movements.

PURPOSE: To keep the spine very supple; to eliminate fat on the stomach and waistline; to firm and strengthen the inner thighs. Beneficial in pregnancy as a preparation for childbirth, by stretching the pelvic floor.

Sit with the knees bent and apart.

Bring the soles of the feet together in front of you, so that they lie flat against each other, with the hands holding the ankles.

Inhale.

Exhale and lean forward, grasping the feet.

Try to bring the forehead right down to touch the toes, and at the same time bring the elbows down, *outside*, not *between* the knees, if possible until they touch the floor.

Hold the pose briefly.

Release the feet and sit up.

Always practise this pose carefully, even if you have no back troubles. If you are not used to it you will feel a strain in the inner thighs at first. Take it gently; if you force yourself and try too hard to get down you will only make yourself too sore to continue and might even tear a ligament.

Come down as far as is comfortable and leave it at that till next time. Gradually you will get down a little lower each time until finally the forehead touches the toes. Draw in the stomach as you come forward. This is specially important if you are inclined to get a stitch when you bend down.

Remember that it is the attempt and practice that count.

MODIFIED SPLITS POSE

CAUTION: Not recommended in cases of high blood-pressure. Be careful if there is any spinal disc weakness. Avoid sudden or jerking movements.

PURPOSE: To keep the spine supple; to reduce fat on stomach and waistline. To rejuvenate the face by bringing blood to facial tissues. To keep the hip joints flexible. Recommended in pregnancy as preparation for childbirth by stretching the pelvic floor.

Sit with the legs stretched as far apart as possible.
Inhale.
Exhale, coming forward, drawing in the stomach and putting a hand on the toes of each foot.
Press the forehead to the floor.
Hold briefly, then come up.
Do not force or strain.
Do not bend the knees. It is better not to get right down than to bring the knees up towards the head.
As the hip joints become more flexible you could stretch the legs further and further apart, so long as it is not painful or uncomfortable.

Bring the legs together for the Head-to-Knee Pose.

★ *HEAD-TO-KNEE POSE* (Sitting position)
CAUTION: Avoid in cases of high blood-pressure or spinal disc weakness.

PURPOSE: A very important *asana*, practised in sitting or standing position (for Standing Pose, see page 92). Maintains suppleness of spine; corrects constipation, regulates menstrual troubles, tones up the liver and other abdominal organs; reduces fat on stomach and waist.
Sit with stretched legs close together.
Inhale.
Exhale and lean forward, drawing in the stomach.
Press the head to the knees.
Rest the fingers on the toes; the elbows should touch the floor at the sides of the legs, if possible.
Come up.
Inhale, exhale and repeat movement.
A great deal more effort is needed to get the elbows to the floor; if it is too hard in the beginning do the best you can without straining.

Follow this pose with Angular Pose, a stretching *asana* that is also for balancing and which calms and quietens the mind and body.

ANGULAR POSE

PURPOSE: Combines benefits of stretching and balancing poses, not only stretching the whole body but also cultivating physical balance and mental concentration. For fullest effect should be practised very slowly.

Sit on the floor with the feet together, knees bent and slightly apart. Take hold of the big toes and slowly stretch the legs out and upwards until they are fully extended and quite straight. The body should be leaning backwards slightly to maintain equilibrium.

Hold the pose, trying to balance for a few seconds.

Come down and relax.

Repeat.

If the balance is bad in the beginning, focus on some immovable point and keep your eyes on it all the time. Another help is to inhale a deep slow breath as you stretch the legs. Stretch them smoothly and slowly, without jerking.

Remember that all balancing poses are 50% mental effort.

★POSE OF AN ARCHER

PURPOSE: To increase vitality, correct constipation, and to keep the spine and joints supple and reduce fat on the stomach and hips.

Sitting on the floor, stretch both legs forward (Fig. 22A).

Step over with left leg. The hands are at the sides, palms down (Fig. 22B).

Inhale.

Exhale and at the same time reach forward and put the left hand on the toes of the right foot (Fig. 22C). At the same time, with the right hand, take hold of the left foot and try to bring it up and in, to touch the forehead (Fig. 22D). The right elbow should be bent and held up and out from the body as the foot is raised. If the elbow is kept close to the side you will have great difficulty getting the foot up. The toes should touch the spot between the eyebrows. Study the pictures before starting.

Return to starting point and change sides.

Inhale, exhale and raise the right foot, holding it with the left hand, with the right hand on the toes of the left foot.

Note that breath is exhaled *before* the foot is raised.

The best way to raise the foot is to put the palm flat on the sole of the foot, and to close the fingers over the toes. This gives a firm and comfortable grip and makes it easier to keep the elbow out from the side, which is essential. The *asana* is called Pose of an Archer and is based on the movement of shooting an arrow from a bow, which would be impossible with the arm kept close to the side.

★SIDEWAYS SWING

PURPOSE: To keep the spine supple; to reduce fat on the hips and waistline.

Sit with arms linked over the head and both legs to the left side.

Inhale, and as you exhale, swing several times over the legs.

It should be a swinging movement: 1-over-up; 2-over-up; 3-over-up . . .

Straighten up.

Inhale.

Repeat swinging as you exhale.

Move the legs to the right side.

Inhale.

Exhale, swinging over the legs: 1-over-up; 2-over-up; 3-over-up.

Straighten up.

Inhale.

Repeat swinging and exhaling.

Stretch your legs and move them about briefly, then cross them in preparation for the next *asana*.

★SPINAL TWIST

PURPOSE: This is one of the most important *asanas* and should be practised every day. It keeps the whole spine supple by exercising all the vertebrae. It stimulates the circulation in the roots of the spinal nerves, increases energy by toning up the adrenal glands and reduces fat on the stomach and waist. It is a powerful medium for delaying bodily ageing and has an almost immediate pepping-up effect through its action on the adrenal glands, which are squeezed in the movement. *Study Fig. 24 A–F before commencing.*

The easiest way to assume this rather complex pose is to start sitting cross-legged.

Keep the left leg in crossed position, with the heel close to the body.

Step over the left knee with the right leg (Fig. 24B).

Put the right foot flat on the floor.

Put the right arm behind the back.

Straighten out the left arm.

Bring it over the right knee and down until the hand touches the floor (Fig. 24C).

Move this hand forward until you can hold the right foot or ankle. The right knee should be wedged under the left arm, almost in the arm-pit (check with Fig. 24D to see if you are correct).

Inhale.

Exhale and at the same time slowly twist the body round to the RIGHT as far as you can (Fig. 24E).

Hold briefly.

Come forward and relax (Fig.24F).

As you face forward after twisting there is usually a sudden sensation of increased vitality and well-being, as extra adrenalin enters the bloodstream.

Now repeat exactly the same procedure on the other side:

RIGHT leg bent with heel close to the body.

LEFT leg stepping over.

LEFT arm behind back.

RIGHT arm stretched forward and down over the RIGHT knee to hold the LEFT foot.

Inhale.

Exhale, while twisting to the LEFT.

Come forward and relax.

While practising, the Mind's Eye should be focused on the spinal region, seeing in the imagination how each moveable vertebra is rotated in its socket as you twist.

After the Spinal Twist, stretch your legs, then kneel down for the Cat Pose.

POSE OF A CAT

PURPOSE: This *asana*, which is based on a typical cat movement, maintains suppleness in the spine and tones up the roots of the spinal nerves. It is often included in ante- and post-natal exercises.

Get down on all-fours with knees and palms on the floor.

Keeping the arms straight, manipulate the spine.

A. Bring it down in a concave position, keeping the head up and looking forward (Fig. 25A).

B. Raise the spine up into a hump, with head hanging down (Fig. 25B).

A. Bring it down again, with head looking forward.

B. Up again, with head down.

Continue this up-and-down movement as long as convenient. Do not bend the elbows at all or you will lose the effect on the spine.

Now sit back on your heels for the Supine Pelvic Pose (Fig. 26).

SUPINE PELVIC POSE

PURPOSE: Stimulates the adrenal glands through pressure in the small of the back, and thus increases energy and vitality. Keeps the spine and knee joints supple, corrects constipation, regulates menstruation and tones up the female reproductive system. Firms and slims the thighs, stomach and waistline.

Sitting on your heels, lean back over them, arching the spine till the crown of the head touches the floor. (Help yourself back with your hands, if necessary.)
Put the hands in position of prayer in front of the body.
Inhale and exhale while holding the pose, which should be as long as is comfortable.

Alternative version

Split the heels apart and sit between them, with the buttocks resting on the floor.
Lean back, arching the spine till the head touches the floor.
Hold the hands in position of prayer.
This version makes less demands on the back but more on the knee joints.

Come up, lean forward and relax in the Pose of a Child.

★POSE OF A CHILD

CAUTION: Although this pose is so relaxing that it is recommended for the release of tension it is wisest not to practise it if there is very high blood-pressure, since it sends blood to the head. In such cases, the best relaxing pose is *Savasana* (see page 36).

PURPOSE: A favourite relaxing pose which soothes the nerves. Also exercises the spine, improves the complexion, eyes and hair by sending blood to the face, and increases energy by toning-up the solar plexus.
Sit with buttocks resting on the heels.
Lean forward and rest the forehead on the floor.
The arms should lie limply by the sides and the whole body be relaxed.
Hold the pose, inhaling and exhaling.
Try not to rise up at the back as you lean forward.

After a minute or two of peaceful slow breathing in this position, come up, stretch your legs and prepare to practise one of the Raised Poses.

POSE OF A BIRD

CAUTION: Do not practise in pregnancy, nor when there is high blood-pressure or prolapse of the uterus.

PURPOSE: Helps to retain youth, buoyancy and relative strength – the ability to lift one's own weight. Preserves the figure, develops confidence, discourages wrinkles by sending blood to the face. It is recommended as a pepping-up pose and tones up the whole system.

Squat on the floor with knees apart.

Place the hands on the floor, palms downward, between the knees.

Spread out the fingers like the claws of a bird. (Your hands are going to act as your feet so you need to make them as large as you can.)

Wedge the inside of the knees against the outside surface of the elbows.

Inhale and, at the same time, rise on your toes,

Slowly leaning forward until your feet are off the floor and all the weight is taken on the hands (Fig. 28A).

The toes and feet should be together.

Hold the pose and the breath briefly (Fig. 28B).

Exhale as you come down.

Keep the hands well forward; if they are too close to the body you could overbalance and fall on your face.

There should be no hopping or jumping; the pose is attained through control and should be done slowly and smoothly. (Study the magic eye photograph, 28A.)

The secret is keeping the legs pressed against the arms. This holds you up; in fact you are literally riding your arms. As you grow stronger you will rise higher and stay up longer, with an increasing feeling of lightness and stimulation. The movement gives a most agreeable sensation of muscular control.

After you have come down from the Bird Pose, stretch your legs and massage them vigorously, slapping them with the hands as though driving the blood towards the heart.

68

Put your hands on your hips and walk forward on the buttocks, with legs stretched and together: 1 –2 –3 –4 –5. Reverse and come back: 1 –2 –3 –4 –5.

Fold your arms on your chest and rock over from side to side, putting all the weight on the hips and thighs.

Lie down, and shut your eyes.

Relax.

You now go through the four stages of *Savasana* again.

1. Relax the muscles: Feet, ankles, calves, knees, thighs, stomach muscles, muscles in the waist and small of the back.

    Relax the arms and hands and fingers; the neck and face muscles, lower jaw, tongue, eyes and forehead.

    Check through the body to see you have not missed any tensions, then practise:

2. Withdrawal of Nervous Energy. Empty out all the inner tensions and try to feel yourself sinking down, using your slow yoga breathing to quieten body and mind.

3. Now begin consciously recharging yourself through the breathing. Concentrate on the thought of incoming *prana*, which is sent all through the body to revitalise you, accumulating in the solar plexus, building up a reserve of energy; and of stale air being exhaled, purifying the bloodstream.

4. Perform the Small Exit from the Physical Body, trying to make a complete mental escape from your daily life. Then switch off your thoughts and keep the mind blank.

    Take a deep breath, stretch, yawn, open your eyes and stand up.

SHAKING THE LIMBS

1. Hold your arms out before you and shake your hands from the wrists, as though shaking off water. *Do this five times*.

2. With arms still stretched, move your fingers in the air as though playing five-finger exercises. *Five times*, both hands together. Drop arms to sides.

3. Kick out with your right leg, *several times*.

69

4. Kick out with your left leg, *several times*.
5. Stretch the right leg forward and move the foot up and down several times, exercising the ankle joint.
6. Stretch the left leg and exercise the left ankle.
7. Loosely swing your arms right round your body, from side to side: right-left; right-left.
8. Lean forward and grasp an imaginary rope, pulling it in towards you. *Repeat several times*.
9. Let your body fall forward limply, with arms hanging to the ground; then stretch up, up, up towards the ceiling, tensing the muscles.
10. Relax the tension completely and let yourself fall to the ground. Relax.

After this relaxing and toning-up the Headstand is usually practised.

HEAD POSE (Headstand, Skull Gesture)
The King of all yoga positions because of its profound and far-reaching effects on the whole system.

CAUTION: Strictly forbidden in cases of high blood-pressure, in pregnancy, to those who are grossly overweight, in poor health, with a history of easily displaced spinal discs or where there is deterioration of the spine or vertebrae of the neck.

Headstand should not be attempted by beginners, alone or without support. If there is no one to stand beside you, practise against a wall or in a corner. Never practise in the middle of the room, alone, until the balance is secure. One fall could cause injury, or at the least destroy confidence.

Never do Headstands after eating or drinking and never at parties. People often expect yoga students to perform like circus acrobats. Resist all persuasion, not only because you could hurt yourself but because yoga is not a side-show.

Never do the Headstand on a bare floor without a carpet or rug – but it must be one that will not slip. Foam-rubber mats are not always satisfactory; if they are too spongy it may be difficult to balance and sometimes the weight of the body pushes the head down through the rubber so that the hard floor can be felt. A folded rug or towel is better.

If you have a genuine resistance to learning this *asana*, do not force yourself into it. No one should be persuaded against their will; but if you are in good health and there is no physical obstacle do not be frightened off by the cautions and warnings. They are given purely as safeguards. If you have any doubts about your eligibility, have your blood-pressure and general health checked before starting.

PURPOSE: To strengthen and rejuvenate the entire body. By turning it against central gravity forces the gravitational pull is counteracted, an important aid in delaying age. Displaced organs – i.e. prolapsed uterus – are helped regain correct positions. Extra arterial blood is sent to the face and head, nourishing the facial tissues, teeth and gums, eyes, ears, roots of hair. Nerve centres and glands in the head are toned up (pituitary and pineal) and the thyroid gland in the throat. Circulation is stimulated, memory improved, also concentration and intellectual processes through irrigating the brain with arterial blood. Increases confidence, vital energy and sex powers. Strengthens back and stomach muscles. Helps to correct varicose veins, sinus trouble, asthma, some heart conditions. Develops poise, balance and muscular control.

Kneel down facing the wall, about a foot away.

With hands in front and palms facing you, interlace the fingers.

Lean forward and set your hands on the floor, resting on their outside edges so that they stand up, forming a little wall, with palms towards you.

The elbows and lower arms are also placed on the floor, not too far apart.

Put your head on the *floor*, not on your hands, inside this little enclosure. The back of the head touches the palms; they help support the head while the pose is held.

Stretch your legs out behind you with the soles on the floor, as though for walking. The body, legs and floor form a triangle.

Take a few steps in towards your body. This raises the hips and buttocks and makes it easier to bring up the legs.

When you have come in close enough to feel you have some control,

Try to kick right up with both legs till they are over your head, with the feet resting against the wall.

Don't be afraid of falling. If someone is helping you they will catch you and if you are alone and practising against a wall, as you should be, you will be quite safe even if you overbalance.

You may not need to kick up, if you have strong back muscles or have done headstands or handstands before. You can then raise the legs slowly, bringing the bent knees up close to the body, then gradually straightening them out until they are fully extended (Fig. 29A).

Once up, hold only for a few seconds, inhaling and exhaling, with head, body and legs forming a straight line (Fig. 29B).

The back should not be arched.

To come down, bend the legs, and slowly bring them down and in, until the knees touch the stomach.

Continue lowering them till the feet are on the floor.

There are several points about this pose that beginners should specially note.

Position of the head on the floor: The part of the head that touches the floor is entirely individual since we all vary in shape and 'bumps'. Generally speaking, it should be between the hairline and crown of the head, but this must be worked out by personal experiment. There is a critical position in which you feel your legs will come up easily (in other words a point of balance), but this can only be found by yourself.

If the head rests on the ground too close to the forehead you will not be able to balance; if the contact is too far to the back, the head tends to slide under. In both cases the neck is bent, which is very bad.

Position of the arms: The lower arms and elbows, resting on the floor, form a stand and support for the head. They also help maintain balance. In this classical headstand more weight is taken on the elbows and arms than on the head itself. It is designed for yogis to hold for long periods and the arms make it comfortable and secure.

Duration: Beginners must ignore references to yogis holding the Headstand for hours at a time. This is not for Western students and should only be done when the body is properly prepared and purified by rigorous training and diet. Hold only for a couple of seconds at first, and even when you are more proficient never more than three minutes. Prolonged headstands should only be done with the approval of an experienced teacher.

Raising and lowering the legs: The slow upward and downward movements are very beautiful when properly done – a graceful unfolding and then a folding-in – but in the beginning do not worry too much about grace; concentrate on getting up, even if only by kicking, for this practice is strengthening back and stomach muscles so that eventually you will have full control and be able to devote yourself to polishing your performance.

Breathing: Full yoga breathing must be practised in order to supply oxygen to the blood brought to the brain. When you are proficient you will find the Headstand not only an indispensable part of your life for keeping fit but also an enjoyable and refreshing exercise. After finishing practice, take a few deep breaths to quieten the system.

Chapter Five

FURTHER PRACTICE

This chapter contains additional Breathing Cycles, Exercises and *asanas* with which you could vary your practice, fitting them in round the essential poses. Try to retain the same sequence each time; not the same individual *asanas* (except those marked ★) but similar types, grouped in the same order.

FURTHER BREATHING CYCLES AND EXERCISES

RECHARGING BREATHS
All yoga methods of recharging the body are based on the principle that individual energy may be drawn from the energy of the universe through deep breathing. It is done in sitting, standing or lying position, even when floating in the water. Yogis also believe that a certain amount of *prana* or life force is constantly lost from the body through the finger-tips, and that by placing them in special positions during recharging breaths the 'circuit is closed' and the *prana* cannot escape. This is the belief behind the ancient *Breath of Circulating Life Force*.

BREATH OF CIRCULATING LIFE FORCE
Sitting with legs stretched forward and together, the circuit is closed by hooking the index fingers round the big toes and linking the thumbs. Press the chin to the chest, hold the pose and deeply and rhythmically inhale and exhale, concentrating on the thought that life-force is circulating all through the body.

Another recharging technique is practised lying flat on the back in *Savasana*, with fingertips resting on the solar plexus. After complete relaxation and rhythmical breathing are established the mind is concentrated on the thought of life-force being directed, *with each exhalation*, to the solar plexus through the fingertips. This is also practised lying on the back, with legs crossed and drawn up in the Modified Fish Pose.

GREAT PHYSICAL BREATH OF A YOGI

Another traditional and very important cycle for recharging the most vital parts of the body with energy. Inhalation and exhalation are accompanied by intense mental concentration on the thought of *prana* being directed to each part in turn.

1. Stand with feet together and palms flat on top of the head, fingers interlaced. Inhale a full breath, hold it while you stretch your arms up over the head, turning the hands so that the palms face upwards.

   Concentrate on sending *prana* to the head and brain.
   Exhale and bring down the arms.

2. With palms resting on the chest, fingers interlaced. Inhale, hold the breath while you stretch the arms forward, turning the hands so that the palms face outwards.

   Concentrate on sending *prana* to the heart.
   Exhale, and bring the arms down.

3. Clasp hands, at arm's length, in front of the body. Inhale, retain breath and stretch the arms downward, turning the hands so the palms face the floor.

   Concentrate on sending *prana* to the stomach and abdominal organs.

4. Clasp the hands loosely behind the back. Inhale, hold the breath, stretching the arms down, turning them so the palms face downward.

   Concentrate on sending *prana* to the spine and spinal cord.
   Exhale and relax.

★ QUIET RECHARGING CYCLE

This cycle, in standing position, should be practised very calmly and peacefully. It could be included as alternative to the Vigorous Cycle (page 40).

1. Inhale a full breath and retain it as long as comfortable.

   Exhale, concentrating on sending *prana* to the solar plexus, breathing out only stale air.

2. Inhale. Retain the breath, tensing every muscle of the body. Relax and Exhale, directing *prana* to the solar plexus.
3. Inhale, retain the breath and rise on the toes. Hold as long as comfortable.
   Exhale, directing *prana* to the solar plexus.
4. Inhale. Raise the arms as though clenching a rod, at shoulder-height. Retain breath as long as comfortable.
   Exhale, directing *prana* to the solar plexus.
5. Inhale, raising the arms and placing palms together above the head. Retain the breath and hold the position.
   Exhale, sending *prana* to the solar plexus.
6. Inhale. Press the palms together before the chest, as though in prayer, while breath is retained.
   Exhale, lowering the arms, while directing *prana* to the solar plexus.
7. Inhale and raise the arms over the head, placing the palms together, then lowering them, still together, till they are in position of prayer in front of the chest.
   Exhale and lower the arms, directing *prana* to the solar plexus.

PACIFYING BREATH

1. Sit in one of the cross-legged poses, close the eyes and concentrate the mind on breathing.
   Inhale, counting six; exhale counting six. Continue this slow rhythm, rying to suspend all thought.
2. Sitting as above, inhale counting six.
   Hold the breath, counting three.
   Exhale, counting six.
   Retain emptiness, counting three.

Inhale again and continue this broken rhythm 6 –3 –6 –3. The slow tempo has great power to relax and pacify the mind and whole nervous system.

Instead of counting you could time the breath by heart-beats, with the finger on the pulse. This is particularly interesting after exertion, for you can literally feel your heart and pulse slowing down to a more peaceful rate.

PURIFYING BREATHS

These are based on the natural function of sighing. Sighing is the body's way of purifying itself, of discharging the stale air that comes with and contributes to fatigue. There are two main types of Cleansing Breaths in Indian yoga and a third is taken from the ancient Chinese Breathing Gymnastics. The HA Breath (page 41) is practised standing; the other two may be done in standing or sitting position.

SITTING OR STANDING CLEANSING BREATH

Stand with feet together.

Inhale a full breath.

Form the mouth into an O and exhale vigorously, in short blasts, blowing the air out by rapidly contracting the floating ribs and diaphragm.

CLEANSING BREATH FROM CHINESE BREATHING GYMNASTICS

Inhale a full breath.

Exhale vigorously, while rubbing the lower ribs and tapping the chest, to speed up the discharge of stale air.

BHASTRICA – 'THE BLOODSTREAM PURIFIER'

The English translation of this name is *Blacksmith's Bellows*. The breathing is accelerated in order to pump extra oxygen into the lungs, just as a blacksmith's bellows blow on a fire to make it burn brighter.

CAUTION: Forbidden when there is any suggestion of heart weakness or lung disease.

Sitting cross-legged, breathe in and out deeply and quickly through the nose, about ten times.

Draw in a very deep breath. Form an O with the lips and Exhale the air in short blasts.

Repeat the ten breaths, once or twice more, but never more than three times altogether – thirty quick breaths. This is a very powerful exercise and should not be overdone. Like the Cleansing Breath it is based on a natural function – panting after exertion – nature's way of pumping in as much oxygen as quickly as possible.

A more advanced method of *Bhastrica* is practised inhaling and exhaling through alternate nostrils but it is not suitable for beginners.

ADDITIONAL EXERCISES FOR DIFFERENT PARTS OF THE BODY

FOR BACK MUSCLES

Stand with arms behind the back, the left hand grasping the right wrist. In a strong movement draw both hands up towards the small of the back, then relax.
Repeat four times.

FOR UPPER CHEST MUSCLES

Stand with hands in position of prayer. With the right hand, push against the left while the left resists. Then reverse the direction. The pressure should be strong enough to move the hand right across the chest.

FOR THE FEET AND LEGS

1. Raise the right leg about 45° from the floor and, keeping it straight, rotate the foot at the ankle, several times to the right, then several times to the left.
   Repeat with the left foot.
2. With hands on the hips, practise hopping with legs bent in half-squatting position, several times to the right, then to the left. Repeat till tired.
3. Standing with feet together, raise the toes only: up-down, up-down several times, tensing the front leg muscles.
4. Stationary walking: marking time while keeping the ball of the foot on the floor and raising the heels. This strengthens insteps and back of calf muscles.
5. Raise the right leg and shake the foot vigorously several times, as though trying to shake off mud or water. Repeat with left leg.
6. With feet apart and flat on the floor, push the weight from left to right side, tensing the leg muscles. Repeat several times.

FOR THE HIPS

Sit up straight with legs stretched forward. Imagine they are the hands of a clock, and keeping the left leg at 12 o'clock, move the right leg round to 1 –2 –3 o'clock. (At 3 o'clock the legs should be at right angles.)

Come back to starting point and move the left leg: 11 –10 –9 o'clock.

Repeat with the right leg, then the left, then the right, then left again. Not too fast. And do not turn the body as the legs move. The exercise flexes the hip joints.

FOR STOMACH

1. Lying on the back with hands under the neck, and legs stretched: keeping them straight, raise them from the floor and criss-cross them from side to side, five times, without touching the ground.

2. Lying on the back with hands under the neck.

   Keeping the legs straight and moving them simultaneously, describe big circles with them – out, round, up, in together, down, round, up, in together, etc. five times, without touching the floor, letting the stomach muscles do the work.

FOR HIPS, STOMACH AND WAISTLINE

In the same position but keeping the legs together. Draw both knees up towards the stomach, over across the body to the left side; stretch them out and down; across; draw them up again on the right side; over the body to the left and down, stretching them straight. You are making a circular movement combined with drawing-up and stretching-out the legs. The weight is taken on the hips, which move with the legs, but do not move the top part of the body. From the waist up it should remain still, otherwise the effect on waist, stomach and hips will be lost.

FOR STOMACH AND HIPS

1. Lying on the back with hands on the hips, draw the right knee up to the body, then stretch it out and up diagonally, and at the same time sit up.

   Draw knee back to body, lower the leg and lie down.

Repeat with left leg.

Practise five times on each side.

2. On the back, with arms by the sides, bring both knees up to the body, stretch them diagonally and sit up.

Draw the knees back to the body, lower them and lie down.

Repeat five times.

3. The same movement but on sitting up stretch the arms out at the sides and try to balance, before lowering legs, arms and body.

FOR WAISTLINE AND HIPS

Lying on the back, with arms by the sides.

Raise the right leg at right angles to the floor.

Keeping it straight, bring it right over to touch the floor on the left side, then up and down beside the left leg.

Raise the left leg, swing it over to touch the floor on the right side, up again, then down.

Continue the movements, with right, then left leg in turn, five times on each side. Be sure not to move the body above the waistline or the effect will be lost.

FOR STOMACH AND WAISTLINE

Sit with knees drawn up and apart.

Lean forward, stretching the arms out between the legs, with fists closed and close together as though holding an oar.

Pull back the arms till the wrists touch the chest, at the same time fully stretching the legs forward. The body should come back only to about a 45° angle, not lying right down.

Continue the movement forward-back, forward-back until pleasantly tired.

FOR HIPS, STOMACH AND WAISTLINE

Lying on the back with arms by the sides.

Raise both legs till they are at right angles with the body and keeping them together slowly swing them right over as far as you can from side to side, if possible touching the floor each time.

You should feel the strain in the waistline and stomach muscles but effects will be spoilt if you move the upper part of the body. Repeat four times to each side.

FOR STOMACH

1. Lie down on the back with hands on the thighs. Slowly sit up without raising the feet from the floor or using the hands.
2. Lie with arms folded on the chest. Slowly sit up, then lie back again.
3. Lie with hands clasped behind the neck. Slowly sit up, then lie back again.

   Each of these movements to be repeated four times and in each case the feet not to be raised from the floor.

CYCLE OF STRETCHING MOVEMENTS

The following exercises are designed to improve posture, increase height and tone up the spinal nerves. To increase the height they must be practised for at least 99 days, consecutively, at the same hour, without missing once, and backed by the constructive power of the mind and un-doubted belief in success. The height of even fully-grown bodies could be increased in this way.

1. Stand straight. Stretch the whole body up . . . up . . . up as though trying to increase your height at least half an inch. Concentrate on the image of the spaces and ligaments between the vertebrae being stretched and in-creased.

   Relax back to normal height. *Repeat at least six times.*
2. Stand straight. Stretch the body up as before: up . . . up . . . up . . .

   Relax back to original height and start to compress the spine, pushing down . . . down . . . down as though to decrease your height.

   Stretch up again as high as possible.

   Compress down again. *Repeat six times.*
3. With feet together and arms raised above the head.

   Stretch the arms up . . . up . . . up, one at a time, as high as possible, as though trying to touch the ceiling.

   Relax and bring the arms down. *Repeat six times.*

4. Raise both arms over the head, stretching both simultaneously.

   Relax. *Repeat six times*.

5. CAUTION: Be careful in this forward-bending movement if you suspect spinal disc weakness. Avoid if there is high blood pressure.

   With the feet together, lean down, bending the knees, and place the hands well under the toes.

   Straighten the knees with a slight jerk.

   Bend again.

   Straighten.

   Repeat two or three times, then stand up and relax.

   Bend down again and repeat the movements two or three times, then stand up.

   Repeat another two or three times.

6. Standing straight, with eyes closed, practise deep and rhythmical breathing.

In your Mind's Eye and using the whole constructive power of the mind, project the image of yourself, tall as you want to be. You must have absolute belief in the method. Learn to think tall, not only during this exercise but all through the day.

Apart from those who want to grow taller, these exercises are important for anyone who spends most of the day standing up: shop assistants, ticket collectors, policemen, etc. The height is said to decrease temporarily during the day. The weight of the head pressing down on the discs between the vertebrae flattens and compresses them. Normal height is restored during the night when the weight is relieved, but over a period of years the shrinkage could become permanent, if corrective exercises are not practised.

THE MAGIC OF SLOW MOVEMENTS

An important part of yoga training, not often mentioned in books, is a cycle of slow gestures or movements designed to develop and exercise the muscles of the body.

An ancient Chinese gymnastic known as Shadow Boxing has its origins in these exercises. Known as the Magic of Slow Movements, it is a powerful aid in attaining the yoga ideal – a body that is the same shape, weight and condition at sixty-five as at thirty. The movements should be done either before a looking-glass, or with the eyes closed, using the Mind's Eye as a mirror, and with the constructive power of the mind fully employed. During the exercises try to project an image of limbs, shoulders, chest and abdominal muscles formed as you would like them to be, as though sculpturing the body mentally as well as physically. The combination of physical movement and mental concentration assists development in a remarkable way.

A few minutes should be spent daily, tensing and relaxing every group of muscles. In traditional yoga teaching there are twenty-four main groups of muscles mentioned, covering the entire body, including legs and arms, and *four* slow movements are dedicated to each of these groups, making ninety-six slow gestures. Special emphasis should be placed on shoulder, chest and abdominal muscles.

The student is advised to study his own physique and to concentrate on those muscles which most need exercising and which have not been properly developed. In young pupils the movements can actually work miracles, literally reshaping the whole body, while in the case of older people they offer a means of preserving a youthful form all through life.

Some of these gestures are given in Chapter Four. Others suggested for practice are:

1. With fists closed and arms relaxed, move arms out from the sides, then bring them in together, tensing them, until the fists cross in front of the stomach. Relax and *repeat four times*. (For chest and side muscles.)

2. Place finger-tips on area of solar plexus. Tense the abdomen and relax; tense and relax, four times, checking the tension of the muscles with the finger-tips. (For abdominal muscles.)

3. Standing straight, clench the fists and tense the whole body, then relax. *Repeat four times*. (For all muscles.)

4. CAUTION: Be careful if you have weak spinal discs, and avoid in cases of high blood pressure. With feet together, bend down and pick up an imaginary heavy bar, putting stress on the stomach muscles as you lift. *Repeat several times*, relaxing between each movement.

5. Standing with feet apart, arms stretched forward with fists clenched. Move the arms apart, as though opening a heavy spring, at the same time leaning backwards with the stresss on stomach muscles. *Repeat four times.* (For back and chest.)

6. The same movement as number 5, but as you move the arms apart turn the body to the right. Face forward again with arms extended and repeat pulling-apart movement, this time turning the body to the left. Be sure to twist only at the waist. *Repeat four times.* (For the waistline.)

7. Standing with feet together, raise arms to front and grasp an imaginary heavy bar. Raise it above the head, keeping the arms stiff and leaning back with stress on stomach and waist muscles. *Repeat four times.* (For stomach and waist.)

8. Standing with feet apart, raise the arms and clasp the hands above the head. Keeping the body tensed, lean to the left, then up; to the right, then up; lower arms. *Repeat four times.* (For the waistline.)

9. In the same position, with the hands joined over the head, twist the upper part of the body, from waist only, to left, then to right, keeping feet flat on the floor. *Repeat four times.* (For the waistline.)

10. With feet together and hands on hips, raise the right knee until the thigh is at right angles with the body, then stretch the lower leg and move it back and forth, each time trying to raise it a little higher. The thigh should be in the same position throughout. *Repeat four times*; then change sides and repeat four times. (For knee joints and thighs.)

11. Standing straight, with arms by the sides, bend the elbows and bring both hands up and forward in a scooping movement, flexing the biceps. When the hands are about level with the waist, turn the wrists down and outwards in a circular movement and lower the arms. *Repeat four times.* (For biceps and triceps.)

12. Bend the elbows and raise the hands to the level of the shoulders so that the arms form a V on each side of the

chest. Push the arms out sideways, pressing downwards, outwards and upwards in an undulating movement, as though flying, pressing and relaxing the spine between the shoulderblades with each movement. *Repeat four times*. (For shoulders and back.)

13. With the arms stretched out at the sides, raise them up over the head, tensing as you raise them; then lower to shoulder-level again, making sure that the palms are facing downwards throughout the movement. *Repeat four times*. (For shoulders and arm-sockets.)

14. Stretch the arms out straight at the sides, level with the shoulders, then rotate them in small circles, first in a forward movement, then backwards. Do not bend the elbows. Repeat until you feel a slight tiredness in the shoulders. (For shoulders and arm-sockets.)

EXERCISES FOR FACIAL MUSCLES (*Practised in cross-legged position*)

To Firm Facial Contours

1. Tense and relax the facial muscles, as though puffing out, then deflating the cheeks. *Repeat five times*.

2. Fill your mouth with air, purse up your lips and move the air round inside the mouth, as though it were water, massaging the inside of the cheeks . . . up, round the top teeth and top lip, round the lower teeth and lower lip, distending the lips and cheeks.

For the Mouth and Lips

1. Open and close the mouth, keeping the lips pushed forward into a sort of fish mouth. *Practise five times*.

2. Move the jaw from side to side. *Repeat five times* to each side.

For Under the Chin

1. Clench the fists, put one above the other and hold them under the chin.

   Gently but firmly open the mouth, pressing *down* with the jaw and at the same time pressing *up* with the fists. Be careful not to force too hard or you may dislocate your jaw. *Repeat five times*.

2. Imagine there is a heavy weight on your chin which you must raise. It is not to be done just by lifting the head. Thrust the chin forward and raise it slowly, tensing the muscles in the jaw, under the chin and in the upper throat. *Repeat five times.*

To Rejuvenate the Facial Tissues.
CAUTION: Forbidden in cases of high blood-pressure.
Inhale.
Take hold of your toes – (you are sitting cross-legged) –
Exhale, coming down till the forehead is on the floor.
Keeping the forehead there, inhale again and hold the breath as long as comfortable.
Exhale, coming up, and briskly pat the face, throat and neck.

SITTING POSES

DIAMOND POSE
CAUTION: Do not practise in cases of varicose veins. Pressure on the legs reduces circulation.

PURPOSE: Flexes knee and ankle joints. Strengthens the back. Used as a breathing pose.
Kneel down, with legs together.
Sit back on your heels.
Keep the head and back in one straight line.
Rest the hands on the knees, close the eyes and deeply inhale and exhale while holding the pose.

POSE OF A FROG
CAUTION: If there are varicose veins do not hold for long periods without stretching the legs to restore circulation.

PURPOSE: An important pose in the practice of yoga breathing because of the position of the arms and legs. The raised arms prevent shallow respiration (when only the top of the lungs is used), and the separated legs facilitate movement of the diaphragm. This movement massages and tones up the abdominal organs, while the position of the legs strengthens ankles and insteps and keeps hip and knee joints supple. Recommended as an ante-natal exercise.

Starting from kneeling position, sit back on your heels with knees wide apart and toes together.

The hands are raised over the head, with palms together.

Inhale and exhale deeply and rhythmically, inflating the stomach as you breathe in and drawing it back as you exhale.

POSE OF A HERO
Tradition says that this pose was taught by the yogis to Alexander the Great during his invasion of India.

CAUTION: If you have varicose veins do not bring the foot up into the Half-Lotus position, and do not hold the pose for long periods without intervals to stretch both legs and restore circulation.

PURPOSE: Cultivates and increases courage and inner strength. Soothes and pacifies the nervous system. Develops mental stability. Strengthens the back. Flexes the knees, ankles and hip joints.

Sit on the floor with the back straight.

Bend back the right leg so that it lies close to the right side.

Lift up the left foot and rest it in the right groin, in the Half-Lotus position.

Place the hands on the knees, with thumb and forefinger joined in traditional way.

Close the eyes and hold the pose, inhaling and exhaling, with the mind concentrated on the development of courage and inner strength.

Practise on either side.

If it is too difficult to bring the foot up into the Half-Lotus, put it close to the body, with the sole resting against the other thigh.

FREE POSE

PURPOSE: Limbers up hip and knee joints. Used in breathing exercises. An excellent preparation for the Lotus Position, also for stretching the pelvic floor before childbirth.

Sit down with the legs crossed. Draw the left foot close to the body so that the heel lies between the thighs.

Place the right foot in front of the left.

The heels should be in line with each other and in line with the centre of the body. The knees should be spread wide apart and brought down as close to the floor as possible.

Rest the hands on the knees with thumbs and forefingers forming an O, and hold the pose while practising yoga inhalation and exhalation.

If the hips joints are stiff the knees will not go down easily. Don't force them; gently press them down with your hands, letting them rise up and then pressing down again. If you do this a little every day the hips will soon become more flexible. This gradual loosening up also makes it easier to sit in the Lotus Position.

Variations (Avoid in cases of high blood-pressure).
1.   Inhale, sitting in Free Pose.
     Exhale, bend forward and place the palms on the floor.
     Press the head to the backs of the hands.
2.   Inhale, in Free Pose.
     Exhale, leaning forward and stretching the arms in front of you, along the floor as far as you can reach, pressing the forehead to the floor if possible.

POSE OF AN ADEPT

CAUTION: Be careful or avoid altogether if you have varicose veins.

PURPOSE: Adept Pose gives and maintains suppleness in hips, knees and ankles. It develops serenity and mental balance and is much used in breathing exercises, for meditation, for many techniques practised sitting cross-legged or when listening to the teacher. For more advanced students it could replace Easy Pose or even the Lotus Position. It is greatly valued by yogis as being both comfortable and beautifully balanced.

Sit down with legs crossed.

Bring the left foot close so the heel touches the body.

Lift the right foot and set it on the left leg, between the calf and thigh. Both knees should be on the ground, if possible (Fig. 34).

Rest the hands on the knees with forefingers and thumbs closed to make an O.

The back and head should be in one straight line.

Adept Pose is practised with either leg set between calf and thigh and the sides should be used alternately to avoid unbalanced development.

HALF-LOTUS

CAUTION: Not to be practised when there are varicose veins.

PURPOSE: Half-Lotus strengthens the back, flexes the hips, knees and ankle joints. Develops inner stability and serenity. It is much used for practising breathing cycles and for meditation. It could replace Adept Pose or Lotus Position. Recommended in pregnancy and as preparation for child-birth by stretching the pelvic floor.

Sit with the back straight and legs stretched forward.

Bend the right knee and bring the foot in close so it touches the body.

Lift the left foot and try to set it in the right groin.

It should rest there with the sole upturned.

The legs are now in the Half-Lotus position.

The back and head should be in one straight line.

Close the eyes and hold the pose, inhaling and exhaling.

Both left and right foot in turn should be placed in Half-Lotus position.

Be patient. Do not strain; nothing is gained by forcing except possible damage to the muscles. You will probably feel some discomfort in the ankles but it is actually stiffness in the hips that is the trouble. This will improve as they loosen up with practice.

LOTUS POSITION

CAUTION: In this pose the pressure of the heels on main arteries near the groins gradually increases the supply of blood to the upper part of the body, but it also slows down circulation in the legs and could cause congestion and damage to weak veins. It is therefore forbidden when there is any indication of varicose veins.

PURPOSE: Lotus Position is the classic pose for meditative techniques, breathing exercises and *pranayama*. The blocking of the arteries in the groins sends the blood to the head, stimulating the brain and clarifying thought, while the position keeps hips, knees and ankles flexible, strengthens the back, brings calmness, serenity, balance and confidence. It is a good preparation for childbirth since it stretches the pelvic floor.

Ability to sit in the Lotus Position depends on the flexibility of the hips, and though a few Western students are able to do it easily, for most beginners it is extremely difficult. It is included here because it is such an important part of traditional yoga; it is seen in countless figures of the gods, of the Buddha, of *boddhisattvas* all over the east. It also opens the way to more advanced poses in which the legs are locked.

The essential point to remember is that time, patience and practice are the only safe ways to master it. Never strain, and if finally you decide the pose does not suit you, you could substitute one of the easier sitting positions.

Sit with the legs stretched in front.

Take up the right foot and place it high up in the left groin.

Take up the left foot and try to bring it up into the right groin.

Both legs are now interlocked with the soles of the feet upturned and the knees resting on the floor.

The hands should be on the knees, with thumb and index finger joined to form an O, or resting in the lap, one on top of the other with palms turned up. Hold the pose as long as you can, peacefully inhaling and exhaling and trying to empty you mind of all thoughts.

At first, even when the pose can be attained in comfort, it should be held only for a few minutes. The time could be gradually increased with practice and experience.

RELAXING POSES

ADVASANA

PURPOSE: A relaxing pose specially recommended in cases of spinal disc weakness. Also one of the yoga sleeping positions in which the body is trained for proper respiration in sleep.

Lie flat on the stomach with arms limply by the sides and legs together.

Turn the face to one side.

Relax completely, while inhaling and exhaling peacefully and rhythmically.

POSE OF A HARE

CAUTION: Forbidden in cases of high blood-pressure. Be careful leaning forward if there is any spinal disc weakness.

PURPOSE: Soothes and relaxes the nerves; rejuvenates facial tissues by sending blood to the face, also to the eyes, roots of the hair and teeth.

This is a comfortable and easy substitute for the Headstand, though its benefits are far less powerful and comprehensive.

It is often practised immediately after Pose of a Child (page 67).

Kneel down with arms by the sides.

Lean forward and put the crown of the head on the floor.

This position of the head raises the body rather higher than in Pose of a Child.

Put your hands on your ankles.

Hold the pose, peacefully inhaling and exhaling, as long as comfortable.

91

★ *HEAD-TO-KNEE POSE (Standing* – for Sitting Pose
see page 62)

CAUTION: Not recommended when there is high blood-
pressure. Care needed in cases of weak spinal discs; avoid
sudden or jerking movements.

PURPOSE: Keeps the spine supple; slims stomach and waistline; helps correct constipation; rejuvenates facial tissues by
bringing extra arterial blood to the head.
>   Stand with the feet together.
>   Put the hands on the backs of the thighs.
>   Inhale, and as you exhale lean forward, sliding the
hands down the backs of the legs to the ankles. Keep the
back as straight as you can and draw in the stomach.
>   Press the head to the knees without bending them.
>   Come up.
>   Repeat.

POSE OF A PLOUGH

CAUTION: Practise with care if there is any spinal disc
weakness.

PURPOSE: Stretches and strengthens the spine, flattens the
stomach and tones up the roots of the spinal nerves, also the
abdominal organs, thus improving digestion and correcting
constipation. Also improves circulation and reduces weight.
The third variation, with arms outstretched, is said to help
cure lumbago and fibrositis.
   This *asana* is practised as the second part of the Shoulderstand but is also a separate pose in its own right, with
several variations.
1.   Lying on the back with arms by the sides, raise the legs
     right up and over the head until the toes touch the floor
     (see Fig. 7B).
        Keep the feet extended; don't dig the toes in.
        Hold the pose, inhaling and exhaling, as long as
     comfortable, concentrating on the thought of the spine

being kept flexible and the roots of the spinal nerves receiving extra arterial blood.

Slowly lower the legs, keeping the head on the floor all the time.

Relax.

2. Link the arms loosely round the head.

Bring the legs up and over till the feet touch the floor above the head (Fig. 40).

Move them to and from you, reaching out as far as possible so that the spine is stretched and exercised.

Lower them and relax.

3. Having brought the legs over the head, stretch the arms, take hold of the feet, keeping the legs quite straight, and hold, while practising deep yoga breathing (see Fig. 8B).

Lower the legs to the ground and relax.

HALF-LOCUST POSE

PURPOSE: To tone up the adrenal glands and so increase vitality; to keep the spine supple and improve circulation to roots of spinal nerves; to firm and slim stomach, waistline and thighs.

Lie flat on your stomach with face turned to one side and arms by the sides.

Inhale.

At the same time raise the right leg, keeping it straight and keeping the face on the floor.

Exhale and lower it.

Inhale and raise the left leg.

Exhale and lower it.

Raise each leg in turn as high as you can, feeling the movement in the waist and thigh muscles.

Relax.

VARIATION OF POSE OF AN ARCHER

PURPOSE: Exercises spine and all joints. Firms and slims stomach and waistline. Corrects constipation; increases vitality.

Sit with right leg stretched forward. Hands at the sides, palms on floor.

Bend the left knee and place the foot on the floor *beside*

the right knee (not stepping over as in Pose of an Archer).

Inhale.

On exhalation, lean forward, place right hand on toes of right foot.

At the same time pick up left foot with the left hand and raise it till the toes touch the forehead. Keep the head up and facing forward.

Lower the leg.

Relax.

Stretch the left leg forward, bending the right leg alongside.

Inhale, exhale and repeat ... left hand on left foot, right hand raising right foot to the forehead.

Lower the leg and relax.

LITTLE TWIST

PURPOSE: This very simple but effective *asana* has much the same effect as the Spinal Twist, though less powerful. It rotates the vertebrae, keeping the spine supple, tones up the adrenal glands which are squeezed in the movement, and discourages accumulation of fat on stomach and waistline.

Sit with the right leg stretched forward.

Step over it with the left leg.

Place the palms on the floor at the sides.

Inhale and at the same time vigorously swing the body and arms to the left, as far round as possible.

Come forward, exhaling.

Repeat.

Change sides and practise twice more.

POSE OF A CAMEL

PURPOSE: To tone up the adrenal glands, thus increasing energy, and the roots of the spinal nerves. Very important in keeping the spine supple. Benefits the female reproductive organs, firms the neck and bust, slims the stomach and waistline, firms the thighs.

Start from kneeling position, with legs slightly separated.

Reach back, arching the spine, and try to put the hands on the heels – or on the ankles if you can.

The arms must be kept straight and the body should arch as much as possible to give maximum pressure in the small of the back. The head should hang back loosely and freely.

Hold the pose, inhaling and exhaling, as long as comfortable.

HALF-WHEEL POSE

This is a modification of *Chakrasana*, the Wheel Pose, more suitable for beginners.

PURPOSE: The position tones up the adrenal glands and keeps the spine supple. It is recommended after the Shoulderstands and Plough Pose because it bends the spine in the opposite direction.

Lie down on your back and raise the hips, using your hands if necessary, until the body is arched. Stretch the legs forward as far as possible with the soles of the feet and the crown of the head on the floor.

Prop yourself up with your hands, which are held under the lower back, with fingers pointing towards the feet. The body should form a shallow arch.

The pose is held while you inhale and exhale.

At first you may find the position of the arms uncomfortable, for the weight is taken on the wrists, which are turned back, and on the elbows which rest on the floor. Experiment with the hands for greater comfort, and put something soft under the elbows to protect them from the hard floor.

★ GREETING TO THE RISING SUN (Surya Namaskar)

This cycle could be included among either breathing exercises or stretching *asanas* since it combines deep breathing with bending and stretching movements. It derives from an ancient rite of sun-worship, and traditionally is practised at sun-rise. At this time the air is believed to be highly charged with *prana* – the combined energies of night and day, of the sun and the air. The whole cycle must be accompanied by deep mental concentration on the benefits given by the movements.

CAUTION: Not recommended in cases of high blood-pressure or weak spinal discs.

PURPOSE: Tones up the whole body, increases vital energy. Keeps the spine and all joints supple, reduces fat on stomach and waist. Strengthens shoulders and arms. The digestive system benefits from the bending, the lungs and heart from the breathing, the nervous system from stimulation of spinal cord and spinal nerves. The cycle, performed several times, is a form of complete therapy and exercise. It may be repeated as often as is comfortable.

Ideally the hands should remain in the same place through the sequence – on the floor, in line with the feet at starting point. This means taking bigger steps forward in 10., which becomes easier with practice.

Note that the movements 4., 5., and 10. are done with emptiness retained; i.e. without taking a breath, so beginners may need to make them rather more quickly than in the rest of the cycle. As you become more adept you will be able to slow down, but you should never retain emptiness to the point of discomfort.

MISCELLANEOUS POSES: BEAUTY

POSE OF A LION

CAUTION: Not recommended when there are bad varicose veins because of pressure of body on the legs but permissible if condition is slight and if pose is held briefly. When practising this *asana* out of doors DO NOT OPEN THE EYES. They must be kept shut and you must never look at the sun; it is dangerous to the sight.

PURPOSE: To tone up the facial muscles, strengthening the throat and root of the tongue. Done in the open air is an excellent remedy for chronic sore throats, colds, etc. Sug-

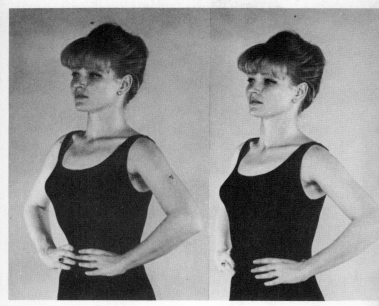

1A and B: Yoga Breathing

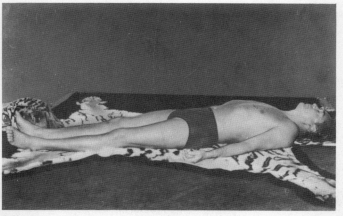

2 Savasana

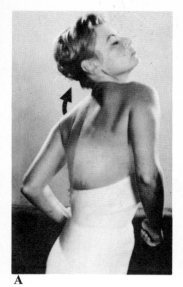

A

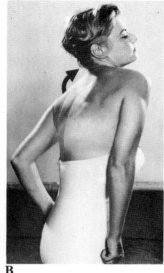

B

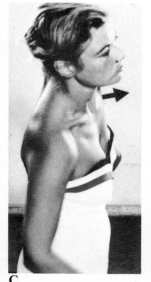

C

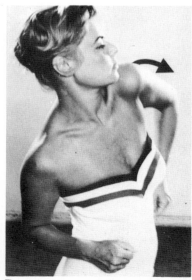

D

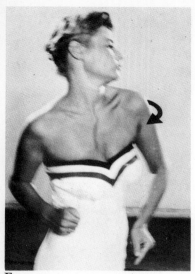

3A-F: Limbering Up

F

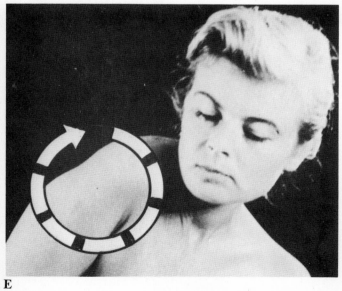

E

4 Eagle Pose

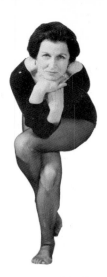

5 Uddiyana (standing)

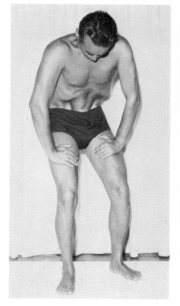

6 Nauli

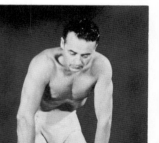

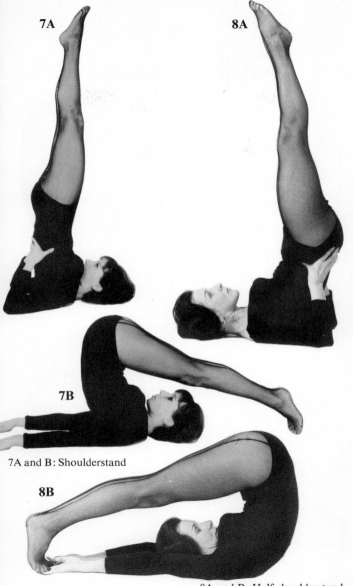

7A

8A

7B

7A and B: Shoulderstand

8B

8A and B: Half-shoulderstand

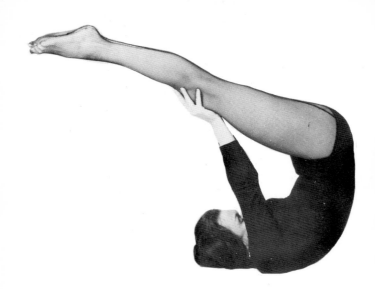

9A Pose of Tranquility

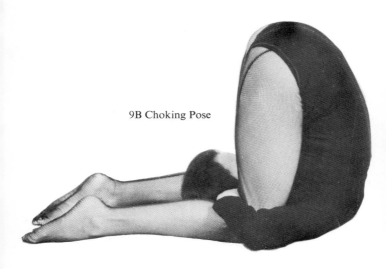

9B Choking Pose

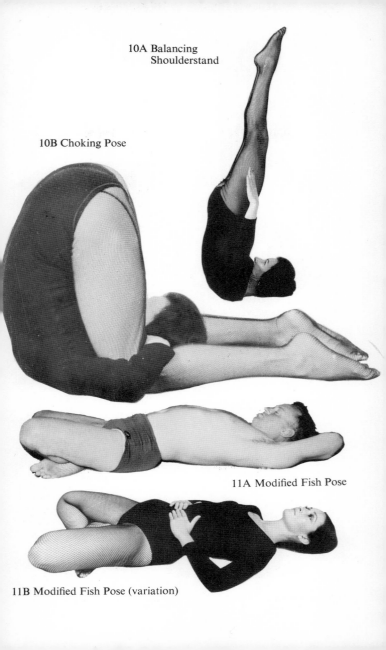

10A Balancing Shoulderstand

10B Choking Pose

11A Modified Fish Pose

11B Modified Fish Pose (variation)

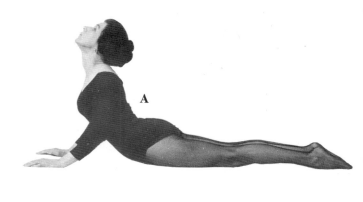

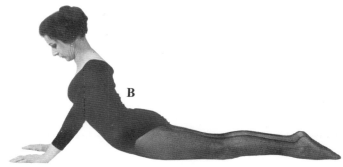

12A and B: Cobra Pose

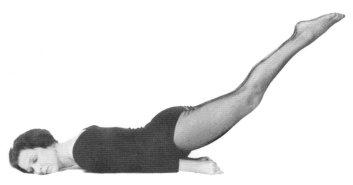

13 Pose of a Locust

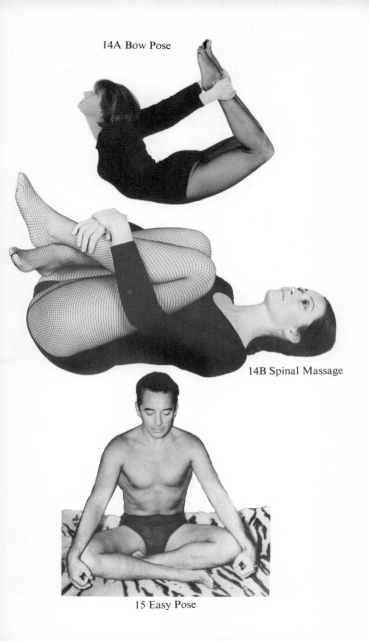

14A Bow Pose

14B Spinal Massage

15 Easy Pose

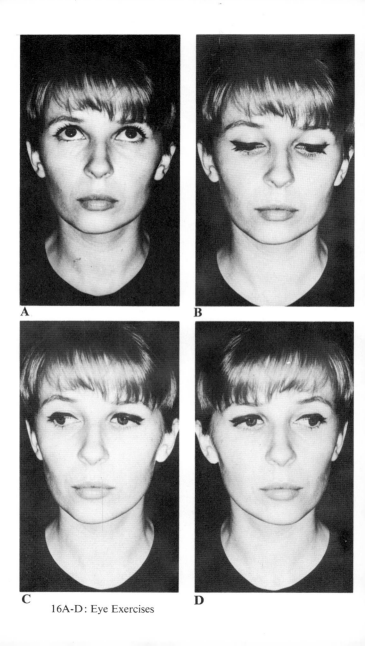

A

B

C

D

16A-D: Eye Exercises

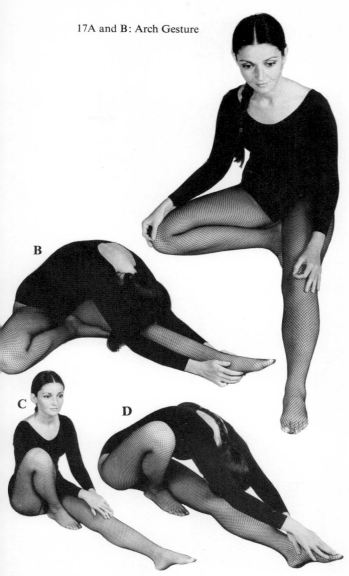

17A and B: Arch Gesture

B

C

D

17C and D: Arch Gesture (variation, ii)

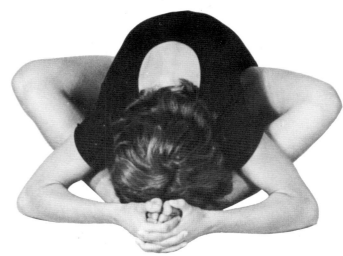

18 Star Pose

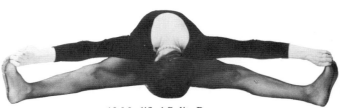

19 Modified Splits Pose

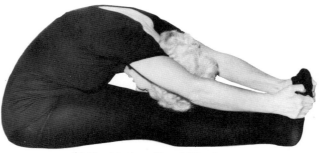

20 Head-to-knee Pose (sitting)

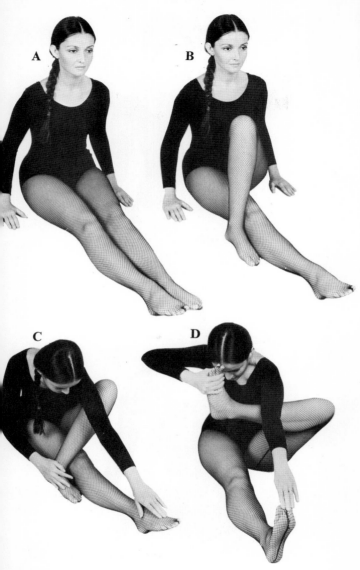

22A-D: Pose of an Archer

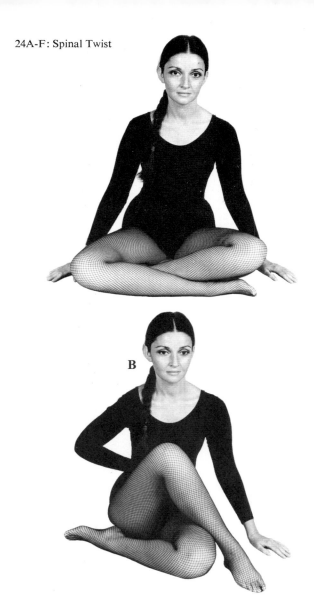

24A-F: Spinal Twist

B

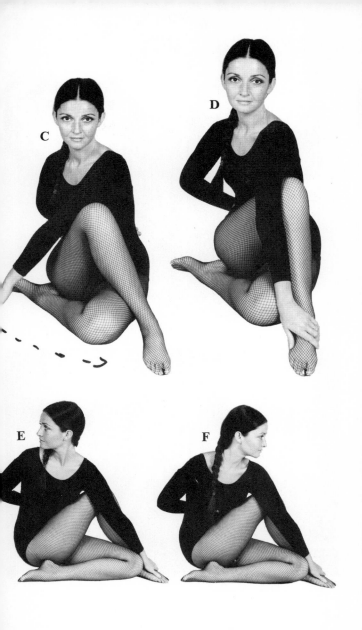

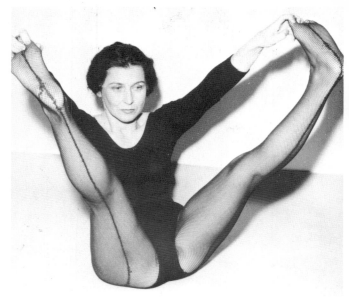

21 Angular Pose

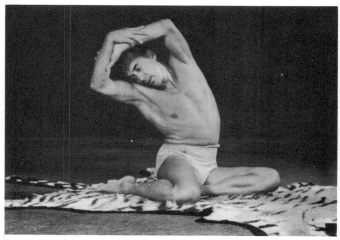

23 Sideways Sling

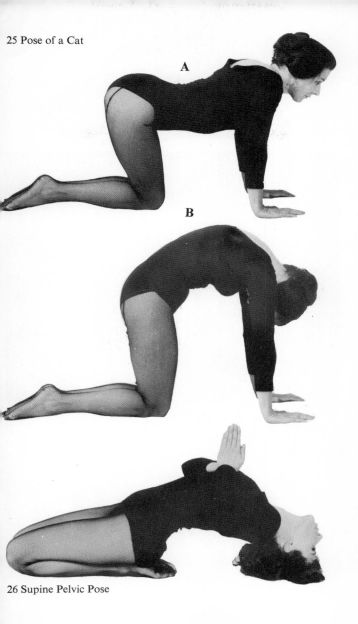

25 Pose of a Cat

A

B

26 Supine Pelvic Pose

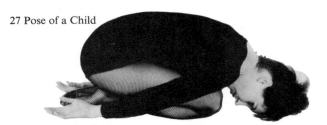

27 Pose of a Child

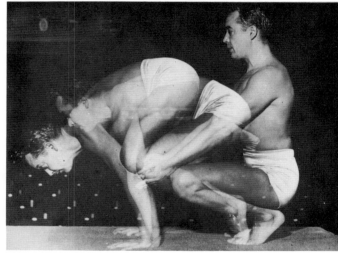

28 Pose of a Bird

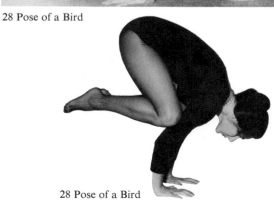

28 Pose of a Bird

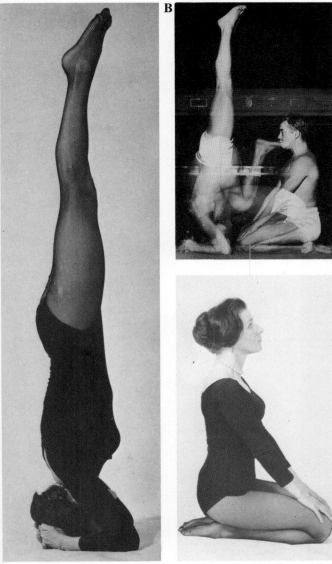

B

29A and B: Headstand

30 Diamond Pose

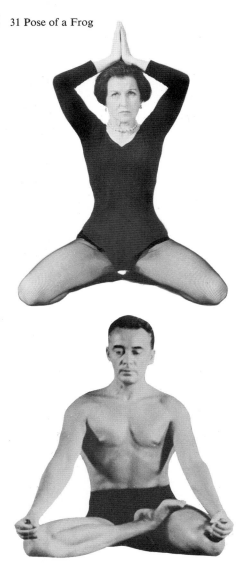

31 Pose of a Frog

32 Pose of a Hero

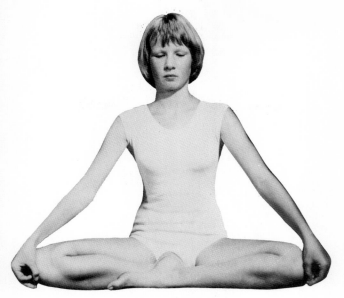

33 Free Pose

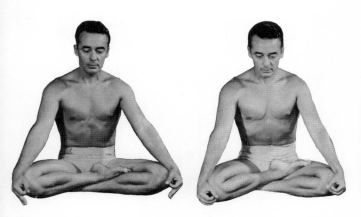

34 Adept Pose   35 Half-lotus

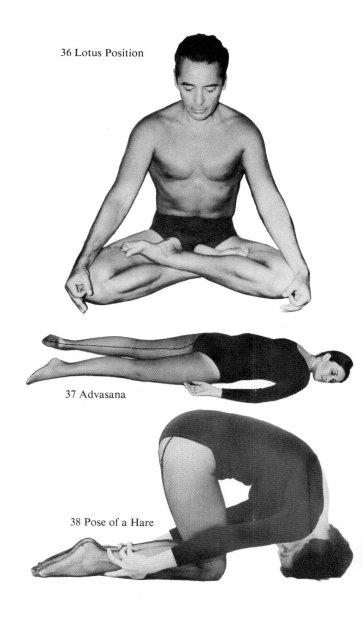

36 Lotus Position

37 Advasana

38 Pose of a Hare

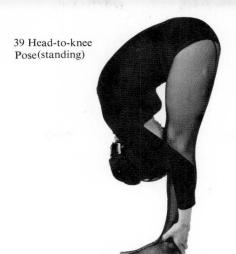

39 Head-to-knee
Pose(standing)

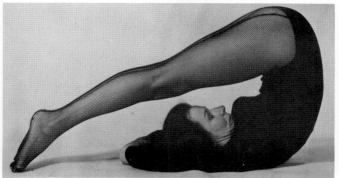

40 Plough Pose

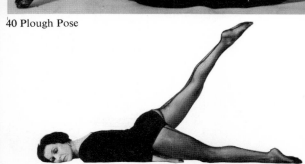

41 Half-locust Pose

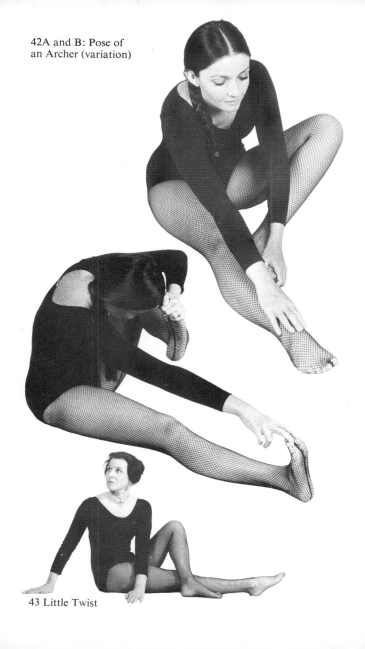

42A and B: Pose of
an Archer (variation)

43 Little Twist

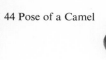

44 Pose of a Camel

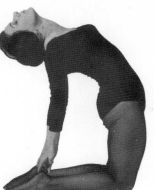

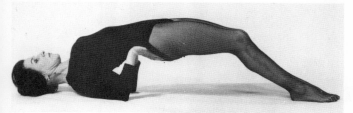

45 Half-wheel Pose

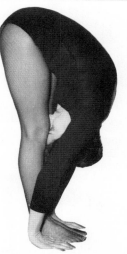

46 Surya Namaskar: correct position of hands on floor, unchanged throughout sequence.

47 Sequence of Surya Namaskar:

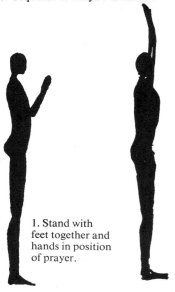

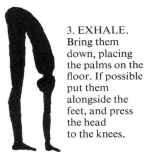

2. INHALE.
Raise the arms
over the head.

3. EXHALE.
Bring them
down, placing
the palms on the
floor. If possible
put them
alongside the
feet, and press
the head
to the knees.

1. Stand with
feet together and
hands in position
of prayer.

**4. RETAIN
EMPTINESS.**
Take a big step
back with the
back—the
position of
'On your mark'.

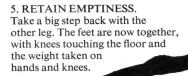

5. RETAIN EMPTINESS.
Take a big step back with the
other leg. The feet are now together,
with knees touching the floor and
the weight taken on
hands and knees.

6. INHALE. Stiffen th
body and raise it until
is parallel with the floc
The arms are fully
stretched and straight.

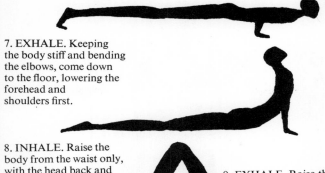

7. EXHALE. Keeping the body stiff and bending the elbows, come down to the floor, lowering the forehead and shoulders first.

8. INHALE. Raise the body from the waist only, with the head back and spine arched in the Cobra Pose. The hands are pressed to the floor.

9. EXHALE. Raise the buttocks with the body making a triangle with the floor. Keep feet flat on the floor.

10. RETAIN EMPTINESS. With one leg, take a big step forward, up to your hands.

11. INHALE. Bring the other leg up so that the feet are together. Keep palms on the floor.

12. EXHALE. Come up into the standing position with hands in prayer, ready to start again.

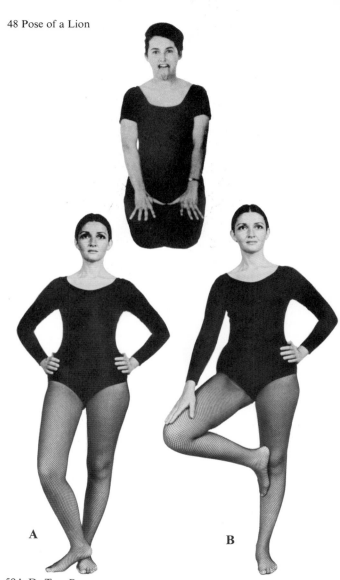

48 Pose of a Lion

A

B

50A-D: Tree Pose

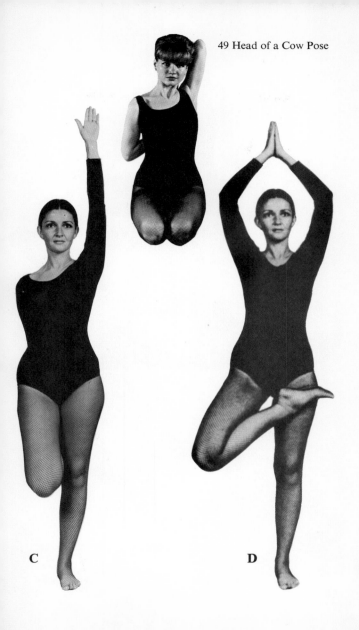

49 Head of a Cow Pose

C

D

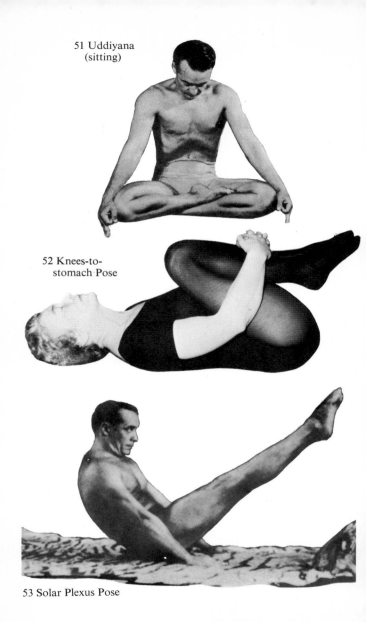

51 Uddiyana
(sitting)

52 Knees-to-
stomach Pose

53 Solar Plexus Pose

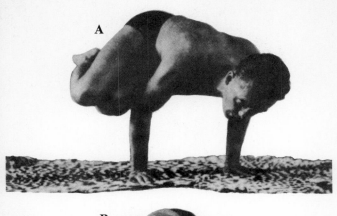

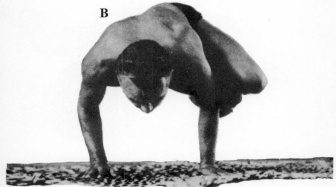

54A and B: Pose of a Raven

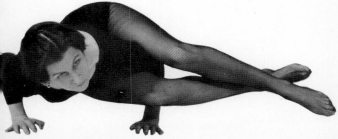

55 Pose of Eight Curves

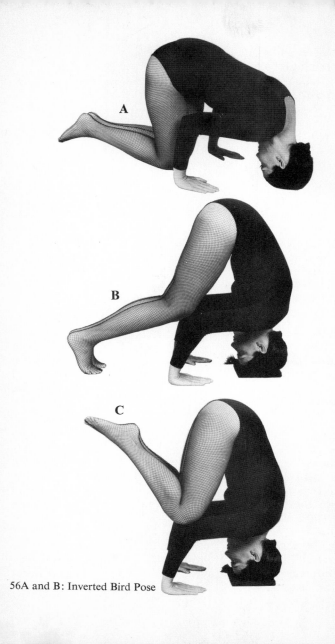

56A and B: Inverted Bird Pose

gested practice combined with Head of a Cow Pose and exercises for facial muscles.

Starting from kneeling position, sit back on your heels. Put your hands on your knees.

Straighten your back, stiffening the whole body. Stiffen your hands, with fingers spread apart.

Open your mouth wide and put out your tongue as far as possible.

At the same time open your eyes as wide as you can.

The entire body should be stiffened and tensed.

Hold for two seconds.

Relax.

After a pause, repeat the tensing, stiffening and relaxing.

Lion Pose is practised either indoors or outside on a warm sunny day. Sit facing the sun, *with the eyes closed*, and when you stiffen the body tilt up the head so the sun's rays can penetrate into the mouth and even down the throat.

HEAD OF A COW POSE

CAUTION: Since this *asana* brings blood to the face it is not recommended for those with high blood-pressure. The position sitting back on the heels is not advisable in cases of varicose veins, and the forward-bending movement must be done carefully if there is any spinal disc weakness.

PURPOSE: To keep the spine supple; to firm the bust; to strengthen the shoulders and make the arm-joints flexible. Tones up the adrenal glands through pressure in the small of the back, brings blood to the face and for this reason is regarded as a 'beauty' and rejuvenating pose. Due to the blocking off of certain arteries, when the right elbow is raised the blood flows to the left side of the face, when the left elbow is up it goes to the other side. Bending forward with exhalation increases this flow of arterial blood and helps prevent and destroy wrinkles, to nourish the facial tissues and tone up the circulation in the face.

Kneel down and sit back on the heels.

Put the left arm behind the back.

Reach down over the right shoulder with the right hand and try to grasp the left hand.

The right elbow should be behind the head, with the back slightly arched. The locked hands will be somewhere in the region of the shoulder-blades.

If you cannot lock the hands at first you could hold a handkerchief to bridge the gap.

Hold the pose, inhaling and exhaling.

With hands still clasped inhale.

As you exhale, bend forward and touch the floor with the forehead.

Come up; change the arms – right arm up behind the back, left arm reaching down over the shoulder – and once more hold the pose while you inhale and exhale.

Again inhale, then bend forward with exhalation, till the forehead touches the floor. (The ankles could be crossed if sitting back on them is not too uncomfortable.)

MISCELLANEOUS POSES: BALANCING

POSE OF A TREE (Each position to be held as long as possible)

PURPOSE: Often recommended as a regular practice for students suffering from nervous disturbances. Like all balancing poses helps to develop serenity and mental equilibrium as well as physical. Keeps hips, knees and ankle joints flexible. To be practised on both sides.

Stand on the left foot, with right resting against instep. Hands on hips (50A).

Take hold of the right foot and bring it close to the left knee (50B).

Bend the right knee back, pressing heel to buttocks. Raise left arm above head (50C).

Lift right foot up into left groin.

Rest it there with the sole turned upward (50D).

Raise the arms over the head and put the palms together.

The eyes should be concentrated on the tip of the nose or on an empty space about six inches ahead.

Hold the pose as long as comfortable, while you rhythmically inhale and exhale.

The mind should be concentrated on inner peace.

MISCELLANEOUS POSES: DIGESTIVE

FOUR MOVEMENTS FOR DIGESTIVE ORGANS

PURPOSE: Tones up digestive and eliminative systems; corrects constipation and indigestion. Helps keep stomach and waistline firm and slim. Exercises the spine.

Sit cross-legged, with hands on the knees.

Keeping the back straight and slightly arched, lean forward and circle the body to the left, round, leaning back, to the right, forward . . . four times.

Then reverse the movement, circling four times to the right.

As you lean forward, push the stomach out.

As you lean back, draw it in.

The idea is to massage the abdominal organs, so make sure that there is enough pressure on the stomach as you lean forward. This cycle usually precedes *Uddiyana* or *Nauli* in sitting position.

UDDIYANA (Sitting position)

Read instructions and information for *Uddiyana*, standing position, page 44 –5.

Sit down with legs crossed, or in Pose of an Adept (page 88).

Rest the hands on the knees with the fingers turned inward.

Inhale.

Completely exhale, and at the same time lean forward, taking the weight on the hands, slightly bending the elbows.

Press the chin to the chest.

Contract the abdomen, drawing it right in and up in a diagonal direction till there is a deep cavity under the ribs.

Hold the contraction.

Relax.

Repeat.

Then after inhalation, exhalation and contraction, practise the flapping movement by rapid contracting and relaxing of the muscles.

Relax.

When you lean forward to take the weight on the hands you will find it easier if the back is slightly arched. The procedure is similar to the standing position.

KNEES-TO-STOMACH POSE

CAUTION: Not recommended if blood-pressure is very high.

PURPOSE: Known as the Gas-relieving Posture because it corrects indigestion and flatulence. Also a beauty pose because it nourishes facial tissues by sending extra blood to the head.

Lying on your back, Inhale.

At the same time draw the knees to the stomach, clasp them and hold them against the body.

Retain the pose and the breath until you feel the face becoming flushed as the blood is sent to the head.

Exhale, lower the legs and relax.

Could be repeated several times, always slowly, with plenty of time for holding the pose.

MISCELLANEOUS POSES: INVIGORATING

SOLAR PLEXUS POSE

PURPOSE: To increase vital energy by toning-up the solar plexus, seat of energy in the body.

Sit with knees drawn up and feet flat on the floor.

Put the hands at the sides, palms down.

Inhale.

Stretch the legs up at an angle of 45°.

Hold the pose and the breath.

Exhale, bringing the legs down.

100

MISCELLANEOUS POSES: RAISED

POSE OF A RAVEN (Left and Right Aspect)

CAUTION: Forbidden in pregnancy, in cases of prolapse, ulcers and high blood-pressure.

PURPOSE: The benefits are the same as for Pose of a Bird: retaining youth, physical buoyancy and relative strength. Preserves the figure, develops confidence, discourages wrinkles by sending blood to the face. A pepping-up pose that invigorates the whole system.

This is a variation of the Pose of a Bird.

Right Aspect (Fig. 54A)

Squat with the knees and toes close together. Put both arms to the right of the right leg, with the palms flat on the floor.

Bring the outside of the right leg against the left arm, just above the elbow.

Inhale, and rise up and forward, in a diagonal direction, taking the main weight on the left arm.

The legs are kept together, with knees bent and toes pointed.

The body rides on the arm, as in Pose of a Bird.

Briefly hold the pose and the breath.

Exhale as you come down.

Left Aspect (Fig. 54B)

Change sides and practise the Left Aspect, in which both arms are to the left of the left leg.

Remember that your hands are going to act as your feet in this *asana*, so they should be kept close together. The fingers should be spread well apart to make the widest base for taking the weight of the body.

POSE OF EIGHT CURVES

CAUTION: Not to be practised in pregnancy, with high blood-pressure, ulcers or prolapsed uterus.

PURPOSE: This *asana* exercises every part of the body, which is felt as a compact and well-disciplined unit. It maintains lightness, rejuvenates the skin of the face and develops confidence. Due to the slight curve of the spine in the pose the nerve centres along the spinal cord are supplied with extra arterial blood and so are toned-up and stimulated. Like all raised poses, Eight Curves gives a very pleasant sensation of buoyancy and control.

Sit with the legs stretched forward.

Cross the right ankle over the left, slightly bending the knees.

Put the left palm on the floor, by the left side, and slightly incline the body to the left.

Put the right arm down *between* the thighs and bring the hand out from under the left leg until it is beside the left hand.

Both palms should be flat on the floor with fingers spread, fairly close together and in line with each other. Inhale.

Move the front part of the body forward and down in a slightly diagonal direction, lowering head and left shoulder as though to put the ear to the ground.

As you bring the head and shoulder down, the left elbow must bend outwards, as shown in the illustration. If it is kept straight you will not be able to bring your head down.

Do not try to raise the legs first. If head and shoulders are brought down correctly and the elbow bent as instructed the legs will come up automatically as a counter-balance. The whole body is held clear of the floor, with face looking forward and hips slightly raised. The right leg is locked with the right elbow and the left foot locked with the right foot, while the body stands on the two palms.

Hold the position briefly, while breath is retained.

Exhale and come down.

Change to the other side and repeat.

This is not a difficult pose; the knack lies in the bending of the elbow. If this is not done properly you will find yourself pushing against the floor and unable to lower your head and shoulder. Keep the hands fairly close together and in line, since they have to act as your feet. Remember that when the right ankle is crossed over the left, the left hand is on the outside; the right hand goes between the thighs and the body moves forward and down to the left. On the opposite side the directions are reversed.

INVERTED BIRD POSE or HALF-HEADSTAND
This *asana* could be substituted for the Headstand, though its effects are not so powerful.

CAUTION: Strictly forbidden in cases of high blood-pressure. Not advisable when there is any inflamation of ears or eyes.

PURPOSE: To bring the blood to the head and thus tone up the glands and nerve centres there. Rejuvenates through feeding the facial tissues with extra arterial blood. Increases vitality, confidence and physical lightness.

Kneel down as for Pose of a Hare, with crown of the head on the floor. Put both palms flat on the floor at the sides.

The arms must be placed so that each elbow forms a right angle. You may have to move the hands back and forth to find the right spot, but until you do you cannot proceed. Without the right-angled elbows the pose is impossible to perform. (Fig. 56A). When the position of the arms is correct, slowly raise the left leg and rest the knee on the left elbow.

Then carefully bring the right knee up on to the right elbow. (Fig. 56B).

When you feel secure enough, carefully raise both feet from the floor and keep them up with toes pointed and together, so that you are, in fact, actually *kneeling* on your elbows. (Fig. 56C).

Hold the pose, inhaling and exhaling, as long as comfortable.

Exhale and come down.

The movement must be slow and careful, without any hopping or jumping, and the balance should be quite secure. Everything depends on the hands being in the proper position so the elbows form platforms for the knees to rest on.

It is not a difficult pose; it needs only a little practice and careful following of instructions. It is comfortable to hold and there is no fear of injury if you should happen to overbalance in the beginning. If possible, get someone to hold you while you make your first attempts.

Chapter Six

MENTAL TRAINING

As violence increases in the world and the future appears more menacing, greater numbers of young people turn to yoga and meditation. Some regard it as a means of escape and withdrawal, like drugs, but others are true seekers, trying to find a way through the darkness. Many go to India for further study and experience. Whatever the motive, the discovery and practice of meditation by Western youth can only be good, and though some might fall by the wayside the recognition and acceptance of its power to help slowly continues to spread.

Meditation plays a very important part in yoga. It is generally believed that in achieving stillness of mind, through breath control, a greater receptivity is attained by which previously unknown depths of consciousness may be penetrated. Though the principal object of meditation is Self-realisation (Identification), meditation on any philosophical theme could be a powerful constructive aid on the path of spiritual development.

There are two kinds of meditation, higher and lower. Lower meditation uses the brain and includes mental exercises for character building, developing imagination, concentration, will-power . . . leading ultimately to inner strength and peace through complete control of the mind.

In higher meditation all is focused on stilling the mind, through breath control, on achieving the receptive and mindless state of superconsciousness in which *samadhi* and yoga are attained.

This book for beginners includes only exercises in lower meditation. There are no disparaging implications in the word *lower*; this form is exceedingly hard to master. The repeated effort required for any measure of success is in itself an important discipline and contribution to character training, while the exercises themselves are extremely valuable as a means of developing mental and spiritual qualities.

As in the more advanced form, they are all based on

breath control and their practice prepares the student for the greater demands of higher meditation. All may be done by complete beginners with absolute safety and though they are best performed sitting apart, in a quiet place, their themes could eventually become part of daily thought, to be dwelt upon at any time.

Always practise in the same place, if possible, somewhere free from interruption.

The traditional method is to sit in one of the cross-legged poses, with head and back in one straight line, hands lying loosely in the lap with palms upwards or resting on the knees. The eyes are closed and rolled up, or focused on the tip of the nose. The Mind's Eye is inverted, all perceptionary senses deliberately dulled – in the higher stages of training they are completely switched off – and a kind of protective aura formed round the body.

Breath is the controlling agent in quietening the mind and facilitating concentration, and the exercises are always preceded and accompanied by deep inhalation and exhalation. It must be the full abdominal breath, with the rate slowed down to the count of at least six heartbeats for each inhalation and six for each exhalation; even slower if possible. (Count mentally or with a finger on the pulse.) The slower the breath, the greater its power, but it should never be so slow as to cause discomfort. With practice it becomes easier and more familiar.

The exercise should not be started until the mind has slowed down and become more receptive. Try to concentrate on the breathing to the extent where you become quite indifferent to your surroundings. When you have achieved complete stillness of position and steadiness of breath, begin your meditation.

Only one exercise at a time is to be taken from the following.

Development of Concentration
A simple concentration exercise is to place an object before you, then sit down, establish rhythmical breath and try to focus attention upon the chosen object without letting your mind wander.

106

This is much harder than it seems and may take some time to achieve. When you are able to hold your attention steadily, practise without the object, with the physical eyes closed and using the Mind's Eye. The period of holding the image should become longer as you progress. Finally, you should be able to concentrate on abstracts, on thoughts and ideas. This may be a long slow training but it is infinitely rewarding, not only in the achievement of inner peace but when used in everyday life.

Inversion of the Mind's Eye
The Mind's Eye is the power to see what is not visible to the physical eyes, for instance past events, absent friends, distant countries. In this exercise it is turned in and you try to see yourself as you really are, without excuses or evasions. If the exercise is to have any value it must be done with absolute honesty but with a constructive attitude ... assessing your faults or weaknesses, not with despair or self-pity but with the hope and resolve of overcoming them.

Inversion of the Mind's Eye could lead on to such exercises as *Development of Inner Strength*, and *Development of Will-power*.

Development of Inner Strength
Inner Strength could be roughly described as strength of character. This exercise cultivates the powers of endurance, compassion, tolerance, largeness of spirit. It takes great strength of character to forgive when you have been hurt or wronged, to face suffering without complaint. Generosity to enemies, humility in victory, the ability to accept defeat gracefully all come more easily if inner strength has been developed.

Fix the mind upon this thought, and resolve to cultivate strength of character. It leads to improvement of moral fibre and an ability to face whatever comes with calmness and serenity.

Development of Will-power
With breath and pose established, focus your mind on the thought that if will-power, or any mental power, is not used

it will wither away like an unused muscle, and that when you really need it it may no longer be available.

Resolve that this will not happen. Resolve to exercise your will, not in the sense of aggression or domination towards others but over yourself; to increase your own powers of conquering moral cowardice, pride, procrastination; to develop fortitude, to regard each setback or obstacle in your path not as a defeat but as a challenge to be met and overcome. This concentration of will-power upon simple tests of character could lead to victory in really serious moral problems.

Overcoming Temptation

The ancient sages believed that temptation could be overcome by identifying oneself mentally with the object of temptation. Continued contemplation of the desired object brings one eventually to the stage when one's own personality is completely submerged and there is such absolute identification that the two become one and thus temptation no longer exists.

This is a strange exercise, which is effective only if it is undertaken with intense and sincere desire to achieve this full identification.

On a more mundane level, dwelling too much upon a desired object could lead to its complete rejection; the mind becomes sated and tired of it and so turns away. An ironic example is the story of the young man in prison, concentrating for years on the thought of his fiancée waiting for him outside. When at last he was free he could no longer stand the sight of her; he was sick and tired of her, having completely worn her out in his imagination.

I am Stronger than Fear

There are said to be seven main fears which haunt man: fear of losing possessions, friends, health, love; fear of loneliness; fear of death, and worst of all, fear of fear itself.

The main theme for meditation should be that fear of any kind is a weakness that can be overcome. There is nothing shameful in being afraid if we do not let it govern our actions or behaviour; shame comes when fear causes moral or physical cowardice. To be dominated by fear is humiliating to man, who should be master of himself. Facing up to these fears openly and bringing them out into the daylight greatly reduces them, and the thought that *all* experience is valuable, no matter how terrible, can help to give strength. Disaster may never come, but if it does we could save something from the wreck in the form of knowledge, understanding and spiritual growth.

For each of the seven fears there is a thought which could act as a guide in helping to overcome them.

1. *Loss of possessions.* All material possessions must be lost, in the end, or left behind. There is no real security or permanence in anything but the everlasting value of an awakened spirit.

2. *Loss of friends.* Separation is *maya* – illusion. True friendship cannot be lost or destroyed by physical absence.

3. *Loss of health.* A good yogi works to preserve his health, but if illness comes he does his best to overcome it while enduring it without complaint.

   Those who believe in *karma* and reincarnation have less difficulty in accepting illnesses which otherwise would seem inexplicable and unjust. Those who reject this teaching could concentrate on the thought that every new experience, even when unpleasant, can teach us something and in some way enrich the spirit.

4. *Loss of Love.* Love is indestructible; love renews itself endlessly; love is God himself and cannot be lost. Though the loved one may die, the force of love remains and so the beloved lives on, in the mind and heart.

5. *Fear of loneliness.* To be alone is to be with God. This is why seclusion is sought by hermits, mystics, yogis. Loneliness is more mental than physical; one can be alone in the midst of a crowd yet not alone in solitude. The *karma* yogi, busy with his work and in helping others, the *bhakti* yogi absorbed in religious worship, the *jnani* yogi with his studies, the *rajah* yogi with his spiritual contemplation do not know the meaning of loneliness.

6. *Fear of death.* To the yogi death does not exist; there are only various stages of development through which we

must pass, in this or future incarnations, all leading eventually to complete liberation and union with God.

Death is no more than a change of clothing. The body is only a space-suit that allows us to breathe in this atmosphere. When it is no longer needed it is discarded and the indestructible spirit is free.

Many people fear the manner in which death may come, more than death itself. To fret about this is as futile as trying to change the tides. We can only resolve that however it comes we will try to face it as bravely as possible.

7. *Fear of Fear*. This is the worst of all because it is nebulous, an intangible state in which you can pin nothing down. Much of it comes from ill-health, from overstrained nerves, from low vital energy. Having eradicated such physical causes, concentrate on the thought that you are stronger than fear, that you are the one in control. Remember that many brave men have known fear yet overcome it enough to perform heroic deeds; that fear comes more easily to sensitive natures and is one of our self-preservation instincts, intended to *serve* us for our protection, not dominate our lives and ruin our happiness.

I am Master of Myself

This exercise reinforces all the previous ones. Sitting cross-legged, with breath established, exclude all other thoughts and concentrate on the idea of attaining complete mastery of yourself; of developing self-control, weeding out negative qualities, petty faults and weaknesses. Resolve to replace possessiveness and hatred with generosity, tolerance, courage, strength and serenity. Remember that a Great King is not one who commands 10,000 slaves but one who commands himself.

Concentration on Universal Goodness

The object of this exercise is to identify yourself with the power of universal goodness, the great stream of loving-kindness, compassion, nobility, courage and unselfishness that flows through the world, despite all negative influences

110

working against it. By attuning yourself to this thought, by making yourself receptive, you could feel you are really becoming part of it.

This exercise should become part of your daily life, your way of thinking. Held constantly in the mind its beneficent influence will make itself felt and shown in your own personality.

Concentration on the Object of Love and Devotion

This is a very typical exercise for *bhakti* yogis ... those who follow the path of love and devotion. Any object could be chosen – a beloved person, a thought, a memory, a religious concept, great causes, an ideal, God himself – for it is the love evoked that is important.

While maintaining deep and slow respiration, focus your mind on the chosen object and open yourself to the warm stream of love that it evokes. Let it pour through you, sweeping away any petty reserves or inhibitions; let yourself be part of it, remembering that love is the greatest force in the world and that it is stronger than death. If, as could happen, the student has no one to love, he should hold the thought that love exists, even if it is lacking in his own life, and that its mere existence in a world full of strife and suffering should give him strength and comfort.

Protective Cocoon

When correctly practised, this exercise leads to mental and physical refreshment. It demands complete openness of mind.

Sitting cross-legged, with slow breath established, inhale, and with exhalation feel you are sending *prana* out through all the hair-pores of the skin. The mind is focused on the image of this *prana* forming an invisible envelope round your body, as though a line were drawn round your seated figure. Through this invisible barricade of *prana* no outside disturbance can enter, no worries or irritations, no physical annoyances such as heat or cold. With each inhalation you take in more *prana*; with each exhalation you send it out through the pores to strengthen your protective cocoon.

With practice and belief in the method the serious student

111

will succeed in building this invisible wall round himself. In time he will even be able to construct it at will in his daily life, when confronted with intolerable situations in which physical withdrawal may be impossible.

Withdrawal from External Influences

It is believed in some philosophies that all manifestations of mind and spirit are reflections of our perceptionary senses; that our senses are the medium between us and the outside world. Through yoga one learns to detach oneself from these sensory perceptions – which even when pleasant are disturbances of a kind – and so make it possible for new paths of spiritual experience to open up.

Sitting in solitude, in a quiet room or the open air, try to detach yourself from all external influences by turning off the perceptionary senses, one by one. Become deaf, blind and unconscious of your surroundings, concentrating completely on your rhythmical breath and the attainment of deep calm. When this is achieved the mind is said to be ready for and open to experiences beyond our three-dimensional world; and even if this goal is not achieved, the exercise is extremely soothing and a powerful means of calming down nervous centres of body and mind.

The Day to Come and the Day Past

This exercise should really be part of the daily routine, morning and night. Sitting quietly, with breath established, the student begins the day by contemplating what is ahead, as far as he knows, for the next eight or twelve hours. He resolves to do his best to act honorably, wisely, kindly whatever may happen, to accept disappointments or frustrations calmly and success humbly.

In the evening, he reviews the day that has passed and how he has measured up to his morning resolves, trying sincerely to overcome faults and weaknesses and to renew his aspirations for the next day.

Chapter Seven

THE METHOD PLUS YOURSELF

The ancient sages had an astonishing understanding of the human body, its functions and needs. Many of their discoveries, made thousands of years ago, have now been verified by modern medical research. They were aware of the causes of ageing and how to fight them, even how to rejuvenate; they were familiar with the curative powers of breath in illness and the influences of the mind on the body; they knew how to attain superconsciousness without chemicals or drugs and their knowledge of the subconscious is now considered by some authorities to be superior to that of our contemporary psychiatrists.

Yoga's benefits usually come more slowly, less easily than those obtained by artificial means; the yoga way demands patience and concentration, but it is the safe way, and its results are far-reaching and long-lasting. We have described it as the method *plus* yourself and explained something of what it can do if you are prepared to let your body and mind be the medium, but some knowledge of your own physiology is necessary, not only to increase your interest in practice but also to prevent injuries caused by ignorance.

Why, for instance, is the spine so important in yoga? It keeps the body upright, carries the head and acts as an anchor for ribs and pelvis, which protect the internal organs; but it has an even more complex function. It is made up of 33 vertebrae, separated by cushioning pads or discs which prevent the bones from grating together and act as shock absorbers in sudden jolts. The vertebrae are hollow, and being set one upon the other they form a long, tube-like passage up the centre of the spine. This is the spinal canal, which contains the spinal cord, a vital focus not only in yoga but in life.

The spinal cord is connected with the brain, and together they form the Central Nervous System, supplying pairs of nerves to and from every part of the body. Sensory nerves report sensations to the brain, motor nerves take back instructions telling us how to act. If, for instance, your eyes report a car bearing down on you the brain flashes a message to jump out of the way, or if you touch something hot you instinctively recoil or drop it.

As well as this wonderful two-way intelligence system there is a chain of nerve fibres along each side of the spine known as the Sympathetic Nervous System. It controls processes which normally function without our conscious direction – breathing, digestion, blood circulation – and which could be affected by certain diseases or illnesses. Damage to either of the nervous systems could cause paralysis or death, and apart from such extreme cases the whole body and mind suffer if they are neglected. Regular yoga exercises keeps them healthy by supplying the roots of the spinal nerves with extra arterial blood.

Since *Hatha* yoga is based in breathing, another vital point of focus is the respiratory system: the lungs, the air passages in the nose, the pharynx, larynx, windpipe (trachea), the two bronchi and all the little tubes and air-cells in the lungs. The chest, neck, abdominal muscles and the diaphragm are also part of this system and are particularly important in yoga breathing.

The respiratory system is closely connected with the circulatory system, which is made up of the heart, veins, arteries and thousands of blood vessels. The work of the blood is to supply nourishment to the body cells and carry away impurities. When oxygen and *prana* enter the lungs, through inhalation, they are taken by the blood, which is pumped round the body by the heart to the cells. The blood returns to the lungs bringing poisonous wastes which we discharge in exhalation, then it sets off with a fresh supply of oxygen, coming back once more with impurities, and so on, continually, ceasing only with death.

While the blood is responsible for disposing of certain poisons, the digestive organs are also occupied with similar work. They absorb food and drink and excrete wastes that cannot be discharged by exhalation.

Digestion starts in the mouth. The teeth, tongue and salivary glands prepare the food so it can be easily swallowed and assimilated by the internal organs (this is why unchewed food causes indigestion). The softened food is passed down by the tongue, through the digestive tract, to the stomach, where the muscles of the stomach walls churn it up further and digestive juices from liver and pancreas work on it; it is then pushed from the stomach into the large intestine, where nourishment needed for cells and tissues is absorbed into the bloodstream. Finally, there is only waste, which moves on, through intestines and bowels, to be excreted through the rectum.

Liquid wastes are discharged by the kidneys and bladder – the excretory system. As the blood passes through the kidneys they filter out poisons, which accumulate in the bladder until they are emptied out as urine. If this fine filter system is clogged, the poisons cannot be strained off and will go into the bloodstream. Kidney failure means serious illness and usually death.

Organs, nerves, blood vessels are enclosed by flesh and protected by the bones of the skeleton: the spine, head, ribs, shoulder and collar-bones, arms and hands, hips, legs and feet. Many of the bones are set in joints which enable them to move when pulled by the muscles, and are held in position by ligaments and cartilages. Others, such as the bones of the head, do not move, except for the lower jaw.

The early yogis had a thorough understanding of the endocrinal system. They realised that these ductless glands could affect the whole body, even the mental outlook, and they knew how to work upon them to improve health, increase vitality and delay ageing. They were aware that, although each gland has its own function, all are inter-dependent to a certain extent and that if a key gland is out of order it could upset mental and physical balance.

The endocrinal system plays a great part in *Hatha* yoga. The chief gland in keeping all working harmoniously is the pituitary, which is in the head. If it is disturbed or diseased, physical growth, mental and sexual development could suffer.

The pineal gland helps the pituitary to preserve the balance among the other glands. In yoga it is also known as the seat of higher faculties, and such powers as clairvoyance, telepathy and clairaudience could be developed through working upon it.

Weight, vitality, energy, attitude of mind, sex life are all influenced by the thyroid and parathyroid glands in the area of the throat. The thyroid is closely associated with the metabolism, the rate at which the body uses up the food taken in. An over-active thyroid could cause loss of weight, nervous tension, inability to sleep and relax; when it is under-active there may be increased weight, sluggishness, apathy and depression.

We do not yet fully understand the importance of the thymus gland, in the chest, though it is known to be connected with physical development. It is most active in childhood but shrinks with growth and is very small in adults. It is also believed to have influence in immunising the body against disease.

The adrenal or suprarenal glands are in the small of the back, above the kidneys. They produce adrenalin, which gives courage and energy as well as vitality. (Too much adrenalin can make people aggressive.) These glands also act in emergencies to give an alarm signal, stirring the whole body to action in moments of shock or crisis. One can feel the sudden tension in the small of the back as the adrenalin pours into the bloodstream.

The adrenals work, to a certain extent, with the sex glands, which are the ovaries in the female and the testes or testicles in the male.

This brief outline should make it clear why exercise and physical purification are so important, not only to yogis in higher stages of training, but to everyone who hopes to retain good health. It might also help one appreciate the marvel of the human body, with all its precise and delicate systems, and the necessity for giving them proper care so they may carry out their work. Even in sleep they continue, though at a slower rate, distributing nourishment, carrying away wastes. They never take a holiday, although they sometimes break down and collapse from overwork; they serve us more faithfully and tirelessly than any machine, yet their owners often give them far less attention and care than they give to their cars.

Even yoga cannot do its work unless there is intelligent co-operation, but looking after yourself does not mean fussing about your health or being a crank; it means reasonable food, sleep, exercise, hygiene and knowing how to accumulate and conserve vital energy. In these matters, quality is more important than quantity. Three hours or complete relaxation do more good than six of restless sleep, and a moderate, well-balanced diet is better than large and extravagant meals.

There are many reasons why people neglect themselves: overwork and worry caused by unavoidable economic conditions, ignorance, stupidity, over-confidence ('It can't happen to me!'), laziness, even self-pity, masochism and a kind of 'martyr complex' not uncommon in women.

Among the conditions caused by neglect, which spoil thousands of lives every day, are ulcers, chronic indigestion, constipation, high blood pressure, nervous tension, loss of looks and loss of vitality.

One of the biggest contributors to illness and premature ageing is incomplete elimination and neglect of hygiene. The ascetic yogi dedicates a great deal of time to special purification techniques which not only prepare him for further development but also delay ageing; they help him to preserve the appearance of youth long after middle age, and to keep his body like a stream of clear water, always the same, yet always fresh.

It is not possible for Western city-dwellers with jobs and families to devote themselves completely to such practices, but somewhere between the yogi and the harassed housewife or worn businessman is the way for the ordinary man and woman. Those who follow it could remain physically alert, active and, mentally interesting, stimulating and serene right to the end of life.

For such people, physical purification means outer and inner cleanliness, starting with a daily bath or shower. If this is quite impossible the body should be thoroughly washed all over; every part – feet, nails, ears, under-arms, sex organs and rectum. Yoga teaches that no one is entirely clean unless the rectum is washed after each bowel movement.

In warm countries people take baths more often, but in cold climates baths are too often a weekly affair, if that. Sometimes the bath is taken at night before bed. If the water is not too hot this relaxes the nerves and helps induce sleep, but morning is really the best time; it starts the day afresh, washing away any staleness and impurities that have accumulated during the night.

During hot weather, cold showers are very agreeable, but they do not suit everyone and are not always advisable all the year round. In very cold weather those with bad circulations would probably never warm up for the rest of the day and could quite likely end with chilblains, while elderly people who suddenly start taking cold showers in winter might, by so doing, bring on a heart attack from shock.

The teeth should be cleaned at least twice a day, on getting up and before going to bed, also if possible after each meal. Brush carefully and thoroughly, both outer and inner surfaces – the top teeth with downward strokes and the lower with upward, always in the direction away from the gums. Brushing straight across encourages them to recede and does not clean between the teeth, which is where fragments of food lodge and start decay. If the teeth are very close together you should use dental silk for cleaning between them.

Toothpaste, apart from its pleasant flavour, is really not necessary; salt and water, even fine sand or very fine pumice powder – not pumice stone – could be used, but do not use too much or rub too hard or you may destroy the enamel. Avoid brushes with hard synthetic bristles, they could damage both teeth and gums. If there are stains from black tea or dark grapes a little baking soda will remove them.

Recession of gums can be discouraged by massaging them with your finger and a little salty water. As in brushing, the movement should be downward for top teeth, upward for lower. And, if for some reason you are without a toothbrush, rinse out your mouth well with salty water to remove as many impurities as possible.

People often forget that their teeth, like eyes and hair, are fed by the blood-stream and will suffer if they do not get adequate supplies, or if the blood is contaminated. *Asanas* that turn the body upside-down, and forward-swinging movements that bring the blood to the face and head will help to feed them, and proper diet and improved elimination will ensure that the blood they receive is pure.

The teeth are also affected by worry, fatigue or nervous strain, which may manifest in toothache even when there is no decay, or a looseness in the gums which gives an unpleasant feeling that the teeth are going to fall out. Rest and relaxation, breathing exercises in the fresh air, plenty of vitamins A and C (found in carrots, cucumber, tomatoes, pineapple, citrus juice, celery and onions) and avoidance of sweet biscuits, chocolates and white sugar help to give strong healthy teeth and gums.

The hair, which is also fed by the bloodstream, benefits equally from an improved diet. It especially needs silicon, which is contained in apples, cucumbers and capsicums (green peppers). The effect of diet on hair was dramatically demonstrated to the present writer, returning to Australia from Britain in 1946. The most striking impression, apart from the abundance of food, was the women's hair. Compared to the tired drab hair of wartime Londoners it was thick, brilliant and glossy, full of life and colour.

Hair must be thoroughly and regularly brushed, not only to eliminate dust but to massage and stimulate circulation in the scalp. It should also be washed regularly, though *not* every day, and when possible dried out in the sun and air. If it is too dry, oil taken in the diet or rubbed in before washing will help keep it soft and shining.

The scalp must be ventilated; it cannot breathe if it is always muffled up with hats, scarves or wigs. Sleeping in hair-nets and rollers is very bad, particularly when the hair is still wet. Not only does it make the hair lank, sticky and smelly, but it could cause the hair to fall out.

All the poses recommended for supplying blood to the teeth and gums will also help keep the hair and scalp healthy.

The eyes always reveal poor health. Like the teeth and hair, they depend on nourishment from the blood and are quickly affected by fatigue, depression, worry or emotional strain.

Good diet, rest, fresh air are essential for healthy eyes. Tired eyes should be gently bathed with luke-warm water and a little boracic. (Running tap water or a clean eye-bath will eliminate risk of dust.) Avoid 'beautifying' eye-drops, they have caused some terrible tragedies, and never sleep with mascara on the lashes. It could get into the eyes and start irritation.

The eyes must never be strained by reading or sewing in a bad light. When watching television let them follow the moving figures on the screen, from side to side, up and down, to and fro. This is a good exercise and less tiring than staring fixedly. From time to time you should look away from the screen and rest the eyes by putting the hands, one upon the other, over the closed lids. This Palming shuts out the light and is wonderfully restful. It should be used as refreshment occasionally in any work that demands close attention. The English novelist, Aldous Huxley, who greatly improved his sight by exercise, practised Palming frequently, not only to rest his eyes but also when he was thinking.

The yoga eye exercises and all the *asanas* that send blood to the head should be part of regular practice and the diet should be one that keeps the bloodstream pure. You should take plenty of rest. When you can, sun the eyes, sitting relaxed with face turned to the sun and lids shut. Gently move the head from side to side so the closed lids are bathed in the warm rays, but *never look at the sun*. It is extremely dangerous to the sight.

Many people pay scrupulous attention to the outside of their bodies but do nothing about cleaning the inside. If the digestive tract is clogged up with waste, poisons will be absorbed through the walls of the intestines into the blood-stream and taken off to the body cells. The whole health will suffer, possibly even to the state of serious illness, or at least one of chronic malaise. Common symptoms are a heavy feeling of apathy, headaches, dull eyes, blotchy complexion and bad breath. Haemorrhoids or piles, a kind of varicose vein in the rectum brought on by straining, is another unpleasant result of constipation.

Regular bowel movements, preferably in the morning, are essential for inner cleanliness. Constipation must be corrected by diet and regular exercise, particular the stomach contractions *Uddiyana* and *Nauli*. These should be part of your early morning routine; it is the best time to practise them, when the stomach is empty. If you are rushed in the mornings they could be done in standing position under the shower.

Full yoga practice stimulates circulation, digestion and eliminative processes, and a diet which includes fresh fruit and vegetables, salads, honey and plenty of water will keep the system clear and healthy (see Chapter Eight, *Yoga and Diet*).

Some people come to yoga to lose weight, but although practice will correct and reduce it if it is excessive, there is rarely an immediate result. If the cause is glandular and an underactive thyroid becomes toned up and regulated there could be a dramatic loss – the fat seems to melt away – but more often it takes weeks, even months of regular exercise and sensible eating to show benefits. Pupils sometimes expect yoga to be a kind of reducing parlour, slimming down specific parts to order without altering the rest, but though some exercises do directly affect certain areas it is general practice that is most successful.

It is possible for the weight to be redistributed over the body so that the whole shape is improved, though the amount shown on the scales is unchanged. This is specially noticeable when weight is normal but the figure is poor, as in flat-chested women with heavy hips and thighs, men with heavy torsoes and spindly legs, boys with narrow chests and sloping shoulders, girls as shapeless and flat as an ironing-board. After some months of practice such people could develop beautifully-balanced proportions and completely remoulded figures.

These changes are even more impressive in young people who are still growing, which according to yoga is until the age of 33.

Figure faults could be corrected and height increased not only by the *asanas* but by the series known as The Magic of Slow Movements – special body-moulding exercises designed to build and sculpture the form and develop correct proportions. Even fully-grown figures could be improved by conscientious and regular exercise; for instance, bust increased while hips and thighs are slimmed.

It is unhealthy to be too fat; it puts a strain on the heart, contributes to high blood pressure and varicose veins, limits activity and discourages much-needed exercise. (Russian scientists have recently declared that the key to healthy long life is continued work and physical activity – a conclusion reached by the yogis thousands of years ago.)

The mental and emotional effects of excess weight can also be distressing. Very fat people often become depressed, they develop an inferiority complex and withdraw into themselves, refusing to go out because they feel conspicuous or because they look a sight or cannot get clothes to fit them. They are too self-conscious to appear in swimming costume or evening dress so they never swim or dance – both first-rate exercise – and they cannot play tennis because they get out of breath. They seek escape in reading magazines, in watching television and in wishing they were slim and beautiful with no effort on their own part – meanwhile consoling themselves by eating more and more.

In youth, the skin is elastic, it stretches to accommodate excess weight, but with age and continued stretching this elasticity is lost and when weight is suddenly reduced, later in life, the body becomes wrinkled and sagging. It is common for over-weight people, in middle age, to go on drastic diets, because of possible heart trouble, and though they may regain their figures they often add twenty years to their appearance, becoming haggard and lined. They also frequently suffer from loss of energy and from depression, due to malnutrition. It would have been better if they had never let themselves get too fat in youth.

Apart from glandular imbalance and 'puppy-fat' in the young, the two most common causes of excess weight are too much eating and not enough exercise. There have been many theories about the value of exercise, but recent experiments show that it is important in preventing accumulation of fat and reducing what has been gained.

Yoga *asanas* will help break up deposits of fat, stimulate the circulation in carrying them away and equalise weight through regulating the thyroid gland, but even they cannot be fully effective if you go on over-eating or filling yourself with sweets, cakes, white bread and white sugar. If you are seriously over-weight you should get a proper reducing diet from your doctor, but if your problem is only ordinary fatness you could lose it safely by regular yoga practice and by cutting out fattening foods. (You should always get medical approval before starting any intensive reducing diet.)

The most powerful *asanas* are Shoulderstand and Headstand, for their effect on the thyroid and pituitary glands, and Archer, Spinal Twist, Cobra, Bow, Sideways Swing, Supine Pelvic all help break up deposits of fat. Also practise the exercises in Chapters Four and Five.

Three non-fattening meals a day are better than starving for two days and over-eating on the third. Regular meals also help you to resist the temptation to pick or to fill up on sweets at the cinema or while watching television. You will reduce just as efficiently without feeling nervy and irritable or looking haggard and miserable. Do not experiment with freak or crash diets, slimming pills or appetite suppressants. Do not try to lose too much too quickly. Safe and sure is the best way.

Exercise regularly while reducing, not only to accelerate loss of fat, but also to keep the flesh firm and muscles toned up. Breathing cycles should also be practised for their effect on the metabolism, which influences the weight.

Do not be depressed by the scales. Bodies with large frames and big bones always weigh more, even when quite thin.

Being under-weight is less common than being too fat, but very thin people often feel miserable and self-conscious because of poor physique. See a doctor if you are excessively and chronically thin or if you suddenly start to lose weight, but in many cases, if nothing is wrong, yoga could help improve a thin figure.

For instance, in teenagers, extreme thinness may come

from growing too fast, while in older people it could be caused by nervous tension, insomnia, an over-active thyroid, a worrying disposition. All these conditions would be improved by regulating the thyroid gland through the Shoulderstand. It stabilises the metabolic processes so that a fattening diet has a chance to take effect. If these processes are out of order you could burn up whatever you eat too quickly. A healthy thyroid also decreases nervous tension and gives a more philosophical outlook.

A yoga remedy for increasing weight is to hold the Shoulderstand as long as comfortable, to tone up the thyroid, then drink warm goat's milk. This should be done every day.

Breathing Cycles, *Savasana* and other relaxing exercises also contribute to a balanced metabolism, as well as releasing tension.

The Pose of Tranquillity combats insomnia, and general practice puts the whole system in better working order. It also gives physical grace, which helps disguise angularity, and the body-moulding Slow Movements will make thin limbs more rounded, if practised every day.

As in all yoga activities, complete success in reducing or increasing weight will only come through regular practice, through confidence in the method, through focusing all your powers of concentration on what you are doing and through keeping an open mind and believing that you will succeed.

Bad posture can spoil even the most perfect proportions, and also affect the health. Apart from protecting the spinal cord, the spine carries the head and keeps the body upright against the continual pull of central gravity. When posture is bad it must strain to maintain balance and support the weight of the skull. The muscles of the back are also under stress, and fatigue, chronic backache and headache are common results. Internal organs could become displaced, causing painful pressure on muscles and nerves, and even breathing, circulation and digestion could suffer. A spinal displacement could interfere with the blood supply needed for the efficient working of the nervous systems.

Inability to relax is one of the worst features of modern urban life, and if nothing is done about it it may lead to all kinds of ailments. Even when there is no actual illness, tension destroys poise, confidence and appearance. Mastering the arts of relaxation and recharging are essential for both young and old. Many famous people of all ages, distinguished for their physical and mental energy have learnt to 'tap' themselves to the source of Life Force around them through breathing and relaxing techniques.

The yoga remedies for overcoming fatigue and strain are simple and cost little or nothing, and the secret of the yoga method is to draw on them regularly, not only when completely exhausted, so that a reserve of energy is built up for use in emergencies.

There are various ways to rest and recharge yourself: through breathing exercises; by conscious relaxation of muscles, nerves and mind; from fresh air and sun; from contact with nature; from sleep.

Savasana, which discharges tension, and Pacifying Cycles, which slow down the mind and quieten the nerves, should be practised regularly, whenever possible in the open air. The air itself, with its *prana*, may be absorbed through the pores of the body as well as the lungs. Air baths, taken lying in the shade, are a restful and pleasant way of recharging. Wear as few clothes as possible, or none at all, so the whole skin is ventilated and the pores can breathe freely.

The sun is our source of life, health, vitality. Cultures all over the world, in all times, have recognised this and worshipped the sun as a god. The Incas of Peru so feared to lose it that at the winter solstice their priests tried to tie it to a hitching post, so it would not leave them to die in cold and darkness. The yoga cycle, *Surya Namaskar* – Greeting to the Rising Sun – comes from an ancient ritual of sun-worship.

In the west, modern sun worship usually means grilling the body on a beach in the heat of the day, which in time dries out and ages the skin, causes wrinkles and lines and possible skin cancers, and if indulged in constantly dulls the brain and saps the energy instead of replenishing it.

The yoga sun bath is taken in moderation and never in the

full heat of the day, exposing the body in short periods to the sun's warmth and vitamin D.

Prana is absorbed from water and earth, even from grass and trees, as well as from air, so to lie in the sun on a beach, to climb over rocks by the sea, to walk across country fields or sleep in a pine wood are not only refreshing and restful but also a means of recharging with energy. (An ancient cycle of breathing techniques is known as Energy from the Elements.)

Oil baths are very relaxing in autumn or spring when the skin is tired after winter cold or summer sun. They are taken after a warm bath, while the pores are open, and the body is rubbed all over from head to foot with olive or almond oil. As it sinks into the skin, rub on more, then wrap yourself in a towel, lie down and relax in *Savasana*. If you go off to sleep you will wake feeling wonderfully refreshed.

The greatest refreshment of all is sleep, nature's own way of resting body and mind. Without it we would soon wear out. Its restorative powers are so great that in some countries it is used to cure all sorts of illnesses, even to rejuvenate very old people, who are put to sleep for weeks at a time.

Yet insomnia and unrestful sleep are two of the most prevalent complaints of Western civilisation and many people have come to rely completely on sleeping pills. Others complain that though they sleep at night they wake up tired and never feel really rested.

Proper rest does not necessarily mean sleeping longer hours; three hours of deep dreamless sleep are more refreshing than six hours of restless tossing and turning. For maximum refreshment the quality of the sleep itself must be improved. Albert Schweitzer, in his eighties, slept only four hours a night, despite the demands of his work. Because of the high quality of his sleep in those four hours he replenished his energy and powers of endurance more than the average man could do in eight or ten hours.

In improving the quality of your sleep the first thing is to eliminate as many superficial obstacles as possible: uncomfortable bedding, noise, light, lack of ventilation, physical and mental disturbances. We spend one-third of our lives in bed, yet many people lie night after night in discomfort and wake wondering why they feel tired. It is not always a lumpy mattress that is to blame; over-sprung beds can be just as disturbing. Each time the body moves the springs give under the weight and the muscles in the back instinctively try to hold the spine straight; they are thus working under a strain all night.

If you have an inner-spring mattress put it on a wooden platform and unless there is some special reason, such as illness or trouble in breathing, do not sleep with high pillows. The spine should be kept as flat as possible. High pillows could also develop round shoulders and bad posture. If you are used to them do not change too suddenly; gradually reduce the height over a period of weeks until you can lie with one very low pillow or better still, none at all. It is not as difficult to do as it sounds.

The weight of the bedclothes can also contribute to restless sleep; too many heavy blankets give an exhausted feeling on waking. Coverings should be warm but not heavy. Bedclothes are intended to insulate, to keep in the body's heat, so actual weight is not necessary; one light mohair rug is warmer than several thick blankets.

Sleep with the window open but not in a draught. Make your room as dark as you can. If you live in a city street which is brightly lit all night put a soft scarf or a sleeping mask over your eyes. The room itself should be quiet and as far away as possible from outside disturbances. All noise is bad for sleepers but a monotonous distant roar of traffic is less distracting than sudden bursts of sound. Sleep with earplugs or cotton-wool in the ears, if necessary.

There is a yoga belief that the position of the bed is important. The human body is a magnetic field and if it is placed against the magnetic current of the earth it becomes restless and could cause insomnia in highly-strung people. The bed should stand with head to the north and foot to the south so the body is not in opposition to the earth's current.

Insomnia can be caused by hunger, also by heavy meals too close to bedtime. One often hears bad sleepers complain that they had no rest even though they went to bed straight after dinner; they see no connection between eating a large late meal, which they are too tired to digest, and the fact that they could not sleep. Eat dinner early, if possible, or if it must be late, make it a light meal. If you know by experience that tea or coffee stimulate you it is foolish to drink them late in the evening; on the other hand a glass of warm milk at bedtime has often helped restless people to relax and fall asleep.

Deep pacifying breathing exercises before retiring will help improve sleep, particularly if done by an open window. In bed, practise *Savasana*, passing through the four stages of relaxation, with slow deep peaceful breathing. Many students have found that they fall asleep before they reach the fourth stage.

Breathing exercises before bed will be even more effective if yoga breathing is maintained during the night. Too many people sleep curled up with heads under the bedclothes, filling their lungs with their own stale exhaled breath. You can learn to breathe correctly even while unconscious. The four natural positions for sleeping are lying on the back, on the stomach, on the left side or the right side. By teaching yourself to breathe properly in all these four positions you will automatically continue to do so during the night.

The method is easily learnt.

1. Lie flat on the back with the finger-tips placed lightly on the solar plexus, inhaling and exhaling deeply and slowly, feeling the movement of the abdomen.
2. Lie on the right side with the right knee bent, right arm stretched out under the head and left arm lying loosely behind the back. Concentrate on rhythmical abdominal breathing, expanding the stomach with each inhalation and drawing it back as you exhale.
3. As in 2., but lying on the left side.
4. Lie flat on the stomach, with the head turned to one side and arms limply by the sides.

Note: It is obvious that one would not lie all night with the head resting on the outstretched arm. This position is recommended for practising on the floor as being the most comfortable, but during sleep the arm would fall into place naturally, possibly by the side. The other arm, which should lie behind the back during practice, is placed there so that the chest is not constricted.

Lying on the stomach with the face to one side is also recommended for overcoming insomnia but it must be done without a pillow.

Although yoga tones up the whole body and benefits the general condition so that sleep automatically improves, there are certain *asanas* and exercises which have a more direct effect. As well as the breathing cycles, the Plough, Headstand, *Savasana* and the Pose of Tranquillity are recommended; also a simple rocking movement which is very easy to do.

Sitting with knees drawn up, put the hands under the thighs, then rock backwards as far as you can, if possible touching the floor over the head with the toes. Rock forward into sitting position again, even further till the head is down between the knees; then rock back. Continue this slow back-and-forth rocking about six times, keeping the movement smooth, without jerking.

Then cross the legs at the ankles, take hold of your toes and continue the same movement, bringing the crossed legs back over the head, then forward. At the end of six rockings, lie down and relax. This exercise massages and soothes the roots of the spinal nerves and helps relaxation.

A very common cause of bad sleep is staying up too late. We are all inclined to do this, to disregard nature's warning that it is time to go to bed. We go on reading or talking or watching television until the moment has passed when we could have fallen into a natural sleep. Once it has gone it cannot be regained; the body begins to wake again, to get a second wind, and it may take a very long time to stop the mind thinking or planning or worrying. Even when sleep comes it is very likely to be one of exhaustion rather than refreshment, such as comes before midnight.

Try to form the habit of going to bed when you feel tired; do not ignore feelings of drowsiness until it is too late. If you are tired but not drowsy, prepare for sleep by stopping work or reading or conversation or whatever you are doing a few minutes before you retire. Give yourself time to slow down and unwind, to relax mind and nerves before getting into bed.

When all physical obstacles have been attended to there

129

remain mental and emotional disturbances, which are probably more destructive than all the others put together. Rows, arguments, grief, worry, jealousy have ruined many people's rest and though there are times, as in illness or bereavement, when intense emotions cannot be dismissed, there are others when they are a form of self-indulgence. Rage and jealousy head the list in these instances.

A conscious effort must be made to put them from your mind; you must convince yourself that nothing is to be gained by going over and over things that are now past and words that are now spoken. If there is a solution or a constructive way to rectify mistakes decide to act on it, otherwise do not dwell on them. Persevere in slow rhythmical breathing, as much as you can, to help calm your mind.

Finally, whether disturbed or not, try to cultivate the art of completely surrendering yourself. There is a very beautiful poem in which Sleep asks the poet if he gives himself to her, utterly, as a child might. When he answers, Yes, utterly, she describes the peace, rest and security she will give in return. This absolute peace and rest could come to us all, if we knew how to give ourselves up to it.

Chapter Eight

YOGA AND DIET

Since the first version of this book was published in 1960 there has been a great change in the public attitude to diet. At that time there were very few health shops; pioneers of natural foods and vegetarians were regarded as harmless cranks, and interest in diet, except for slimming, was considered eccentric unless you were ill or observed religious dietary laws. Young people in particular avoided the food that could do them most good.

We now have health shops in every suburb and town, health and vegetarian restaurants flourish, 'health foods' are sold even in supermarkets, and people drive miles in search of organically-grown fresh fruit and vegetables. It is quite common for city health bars to be crowded at midday with teenagers queuing up for fruit juice or yoghurt or salads; at weekends young girls lunching away from home go out to buy foods they would have rejected ten years before. Increasing numbers of women are making their own bread from stone-ground wholemeal flour and many people have become partly or completely vegetarian.

Publicity about pollution and the dangers of chemical fertilisers has brought a realisation of how far removed we are from a natural way of living and inspired a healthy desire to do something about it before it is too late.

Some young yoga enthusiasts even try to live on the traditional yoga diet. This is lacto-vegetarian and in India would probably be curds, *ghee* or clarified butter, vegetables, perhaps berries and roots from the forest. India is a country with great poverty and the average Indian has never been used to rich or elaborate meals; even so, the yogi's diet is extremely sparse. He is completely vegetarian, partly for reasons of purification and also because he does not wish to take life. He eats only *sattvic* foods, which are mild, not stimulating or highly-flavoured, to cultivate *Sattva* the Shining, the happiness of enlightenment and understanding, and to discourage such destructive instincts as hatred, rage and violence.

Such a diet is not suitable for active people living an urban working life. In fact, it is not unusual for Western disciples to find the food of Indian *ashrams* inadequate, even to become ill until they can adapt to it.

Europeans can be good yoga students without extreme austerities. In the *Bhagavad-Gita* the yogi is told to be moderate in eating and recreation, moderately active, moderate in sleep; in short, to use commonsense. The householder yogi's main concern should be to nourish his body as wisely as possible, to avoid excesses and all forms of poisoning, neither overeating in general nor taking too much of any one thing; not poisoning his system with alcohol, nicotine, drugs or the slow chronic contamination of a sluggish eliminative system.

The main principles for guidance should be Selectivity, Moderation and proper Mastication.

Selectivity means choosing only pure foods, to reduce all possible inner pollution. Diet is a very individual affair; people's requirements vary according to the work they do and the amount of energy they use up. Everyone should study his own personal needs and biological type so that by the time he reaches middle age he has a good idea of what foods suit him best.

All middle-aged people should watch their diet and avoid foods that do little beyond putting on weight. As we get older we should eat less, particularly of animal fats, for the body no longer burns it up as in more active youth and the result is increased weight and possible damage to health.

Warnings about coronary occlusions have confused many people. One year they are told to avoid certain foods, the next something else is forbidden. If you are worried, have your blood tested for cholesterol and, if all is well, keep to a normal well-balanced diet. If cholesterol is too high your doctor will prescribe a diet to reduce it. He will probably also advise exercise and usually yoga is the most suitable, so long as any cautions and prohibitions given are observed. (At the time of writing the medical world is still unsure if cholesterol is really the cause of coronary occlusions.)

The French gastronome, Brillat-Savarin, wrote, 'Tell me what you eat and I will tell you who you are', but many people need not tell what they eat; it shows clearly in their appearance. Gluttons are overweight, with blotchy complexions, lethargic and irritable because of sluggish livers and bad digestions, while malnutrition gives a haggard and drawn appearance, a depressed and listless air.

Yoga teaches that weight and measurements should be more or less the same all through life. The body should be moulded into its final form by the age of 33 and from then there should be little change. A slight increase is permitted in middle age but after that the former weight should be regained and preserved. Not many people keep to this rule. Most have lost their figures long before they reach forty.

In working out your personal diet, make use of modern knowledge and of the wisdom of the past, including items recommended by centuries of experience yet profiting from an understanding of calorie values.

A sensible diet for normal Western students should include fruit, vegetables, milk or milk products – butter, cheese, yoghurt or buttermilk – eggs, honey, nuts, fish and meat in moderation if desired. The present ban on eggs and milk products because of cholesterol (which could be changed tomorrow) must be interpreted with commonsense according to your own health and your doctor's advice.

White bread and white sugar should be replaced by wholemeal bread and honey. Honey, dates, fruit or fruit-juices will supply the sugar we need for good health. A spoonful of honey at breakfast every day not only provides energy, it also improves health and appearance and gradually reduces the craving for sweets or cakes.

If you have been brought up to eat meat there is no need to suddenly give it up completely, though there is no doubt that for some a good vegetarian diet is best. It can be completely nourishing; there have been outstanding athletes and fine physical specimens who have never touched meat, and many strong animals – the horse, ox, gorilla, elephant – are not carnivorous.

Apart from the question of taking life, a meat diet is abhorrent to many vegetarians since it means eating a corpse

133

in the very first stages of decomposition. A short meditation on this could help destroy an appetite for animal flesh.

Vegetarian meals are now far pleasanter than they used to be; they no longer need be depressing affairs of boiled vegetables and cold grated carrot. There are plenty of interesting vegetarian cookery books and much can be learnt about meatless meals from other countries. In China and Japan, vegetables are given the minimum of cooking and so retain high nutritional content and maximum flavour; Turkey has meatless *pilaffs*, meatless stews and casseroles, stuffed vineleaves, stuffed vegetables of all sorts; Russia has meatless soups, some made from fruit, salads and cheese and meatless *zakuski* (hors d'oeuvres); India has vegetable curries. All these countries use rice, which they cook in interesting ways, and all use fresh fruit whenever available. Vegetarian meals, like any others, depend on the cook's ability and imagination, and when properly prepared they are so good that the absence of meat is not noticed.

Moderation is the second important principle in diet. Most people overeat and even when not at table are constantly picking or having snacks between meals. You should eat only when you are hungry, and try to have regular meals. If children and teenagers, who usually have big appetites, are hungry between meals train them to eat cheese, fruit – dried or fresh – even raw vegetables like carrots and radishes instead of biscuits and cakes.

Keep meals simple, not eating too many different foods all together. The fact that many people have digestive upsets after parties suggests that too much all at once upsets the metabolic balance.

Do not be influenced by fashions or fads, or by women's magazine and newspaper supplements that fill up their pages with endless 'new' ideas about food, mostly quite useless and often without nutritional value. The different slimming or so-called health diets suggested every week may not be universally suitable; all constitutions cannot tolerate a diet almost entirely made up of eggs, for instance, or vast quantities of apple-cider vinegar.

Fried and heated-up foods are best avoided, particularly when digestion is poor. If you must fry – e.g. an occasional omelette – use a minimum of oil, polyunsaturated, if necessary.

Mastication is the third important rule. Chew everything thoroughly and remember that digestion begins in the mouth. Eating heavily when you are overtired, in a bad temper or emotionally upset usually gives indigestion, and as already mentioned, large meals late at night can cause insomnia.

All this does not mean one should be obsessed with digestion or turn meals into solemn silent occasions. Even when alone they should be a pleasant event, eaten in an agreeable relaxed frame of mind. If you have company, talk while you eat; enjoy yourself. Conversation and laughter are excellent for the digestion.

Ideal conditions are not always possible but often there could be improvements. Getting up a little earlier or spending less time before the mirror could make breakfast much pleasanter. The usual Western breakfast is a hasty snatch at something as you stand at the stove or run for the bus. If you have a large breakfast in a hurry you are bound to pay for it. Bacon and eggs eaten under hurried conditions will feel like lead in your stomach.

In a world where millions die of hunger every yeat, many people still sit down each morning to chops, steak and sausages; many still eat meat three times a day, particularly in Australia and Argentina, both meat-producing countries, and both with a hot summer in which such a heavy diet is most unhealthy.

An ideal summer breakfast, which could also be taken all the year round, is yoghurt with fresh or stewed fruit and honey. Fresh fruit juice, wholemeal bread or toast and honey and whatever you normally have for a hot drink makes a nourishing and easily digested breakfast.

Meat once a day is more than enough, even three times a week could be adequate. Grill it whenever possible and if cooking joints use oil instead of dripping. Meat, with fat trimmed off, slowly cooked in a casserole with vegetables, fish, fresh salads and fruit are all good and do not increase the weight. Even in winter, eat a green salad after the main course and serve fruit with cheese instead of sweet or heavy puddings.

Apart from salads, as many vegetables as possible could be eaten raw, and in any case should never be overcooked. Steam them or use the minimum of water. Do not let them stand in it, before or after cooking. Any cooking liquid left should be kept for stock and put into soup.

In winter it is a good idea to have a regular supply of soups or vegetable consommé available. Keep it in the refrigerator overnight, if the kitchen is warm, and boil it up before eating.

In summer, drink the juice of fresh fruit, if necessary sweetened with honey. If you have your own juice extractor it will enable you to make these drinks whenever you want them. The best drink of all is water, the cheapest and, in the West, the easiest to obtain. Drink as much of it as you can, between meals, to flush out the kidneys, but do not gulp it down with food. Cold water with hot meat or fresh bread gives a horribly bloated feeling.

Nothing should ever be gulped, particularly milk. Milk is an important food as well as a drink and should be 'chewed' and swallowed slowly. Unfortunately it does not suit everyone so if it disagrees with you or is forbidden because of fat content try cultured buttermilk, or the mixture known in Turkey as *ayran*. This is a remarkable drink, light, nourishing, digestible and very easily made. Beat together equal quantities of plain yoghurt and water, with a pinch of salt, and drink it cold.

Yoghurt itself is a very good food and so popular one would think it needed no comment; yet commercial yoghurt, which contains gelatine, sugar, fruit flavours and colouring, bears little relation to the real product. The added sweetness makes it useless for slimming diets. True yoghurt has a runny consistency and is not at all sweet; its flavour is rather sharp and may not appeal at first, but the taste is soon acquired and enjoyed – like getting used to tea without sugar.

If proper yoghurt is not available you could try making your own. In Turkey, where it is used constantly with meat, vegetables, in cooking and as a sauce, most housewives make it fresh every day, The method is rather like making Devonshire cream.

136

You need either the bacillus for starting the yoghurt, which you could buy from a health food shop, or a small amount of left-over *real* yoghurt, not the sweetened gelatine mixture. Pour the milk – goat or cow – into a wide shallow basin (a Devonshire milk pan is ideal), and let it stand overnight in a reasonably warm place; not on a stove or by a heater, just at normal room temperature. This allows the cream to rise to the top. In the morning, put in the bacillus or a teaspoon of yesterday's yoghurt and leave in a warm place all day and during the night. In the morning your yoghurt is ready for breakfast.

Some people stand the bowl in a sunny window, though not in the direct sunlight. At first you may have to experiment with temperatures and quantities but the process is so simple you will soon master it. It will not be a smooth and solid consistency like commercial yoghurt; it will be more liquid and perhaps rather lumpy, but it will be the real thing. Keep a little aside for next day's batch and repeat the process as long as you like.

Though *fasting* is a well-known feature of yoga training, authorities do not always agree about it. Some believe it is essential, others say that a proper yoga diet makes it unnecessary. It is claimed that fasting was condemned by the ancient sages as bad for the health, that the *Gita* itself says yoga is not for the man who fasts excessively. But whatever views are held on its physical value, traditionally it has always been practised in East and West by saints, mystics and yogis for spiritual purification.

On the physical plane, to fast is to go without food voluntarily, in order to help the body throw off poisons or impurities. This is not the same as starving, which is a destructive process and not usually undertaken willingly – except perhaps in extreme cases, such as hunger strikes for achieving some aim. Starving is not natural, whereas occasional fasting is. Animals fast when they are sick and the human body rejects food in illness. It is nature's way of conserving all energies in the fight for recovery.

Long fasts are not suitable for ordinary Europeans living busy lives. Short or partial fasts are quite adequate and even these should be practised with commonsense. They should not be observed at all by anyone who is very much under-weight or suffering from anaemia or in a low state of health, and should be forbidden to children who are still growing. If you want to fast but are unsure if it is right for you, you should ask your doctor's advice.

Assuming that you are in normal health and strength, it is a good plan, in the spring, to have a day when nothing is taken but water and fruit juices, or several days when only fruit is eaten. You could even fast completely for a day or so if it can be done at a time when no demands are being made on you, when you can take plenty of rest and go to bed early. It should not last for more than two days. An enema each evening, to help get rid of impurities, is part of traditional practice.

A day of complete silence is also very refreshing, resting the whole system and conserving all possible energy. It is best to not even read, since using the eyes takes up vitality.

A form of partial fasting known as *Seasonal Purification* is done at the change of the year, using natural foods available at these times. Spring is the best season, not only because it leads into summer, when life is generally easier and pleasanter, but also because this is a time of rejuvenation in nature. An ancient instinct makes us want to share in this revitalising period, to make a fresh start in different ways, even if only spring-cleaning the house; and the body could also be ready for spring-cleaning after a heavy winter diet.

Like all other fasts, *Seasonal Purification* is done with care, taking all possible rest and sleep and avoiding undue strain and exertion. For one week – traditionally the first week of spring – observe the following regime:

First Day: Complete water fast. No food at all to be taken. Nothing to drink but water, but plenty of it. No tea or coffee, with or without milk. An enema before going to bed is recommended.

Second Day: Only fruit juice to be drunk. It may be what fruit you like so long as it is all the same. No mixtures, no sweetening.

Third Day: Eating is allowed but only fruit, and it must be all

138

of the same kind: either all citrus or all stone fruits. For instance, you may have grapefruit, orange and mandarin, or peaches, plums and apricots, but not oranges, peaches and bananas; (it is also not advisable to eat only bananas all day). *Fourth, fifth, sixth, seventh days:* Eat a four-ingredient diet of fruit, vegetables, honey and nuts. They may be mixed but do not eat too much of anything. The maximum calories each day should be 1000.

After this week, if you have followed instructions and taken plenty of rest, you will feel light, well and refreshed. Do as many breathing and recharging exercises as possible, ideally in the open air, or at least by an open window. If you are on holiday or if you do not go to work, take sun baths, air baths and oil baths. Relax as much as you can in the open air.

In breaking a fast, be careful not to start with large heavy meals, no matter how hungry you feel. Begin gradually with fruit juice, fruit, vegetables or vegetable consommé, and drink plenty of water.

Sometimes people claim to be upset by fasting when it is really the resumption of eating that has caused the trouble. The digestive system needs time to adapt after the absence of food and must not be hurried or forced. Victims of starvation are never allowed heavy meals at first; in extreme cases they have even died from eating too much, too suddenly.

Inner contamination through constipation, discussed in the last chapter, is the most common form of bodily poisoning and one that can exist unsuspected for years. Though you have a bowel movement each day you could still suffer from incomplete elimination, if the system is sluggish, and consequently from internal poisoning.

To cure constipation, as well as the exercises recommended and the daily practice of abdominal contractions, the diet should be adjusted. Avoid heavy starch meals, take plenty of fruit, fruit juice, green salads and vegetables. Regular relaxation is also important; it is well-known that mental and emotional strain can bring on diarrhoea and stomach upsets but not always realised that it can also cause constipation.

Tobacco, alcohol and drugs are unacceptable to yoga. Students who smoke do so without their teacher's approval. Since the whole system of training is based on breathing and designed to increase the supply of fresh air in the lungs it is unlikely that it could condone a practice which, if it does nothing worse, lines delicate membranes and tissues with thick black tar.

No one with any respect for his body would be a heavy smoker. Many people, alarmed by talk of lung cancer, have tried to break the habit and some have succeeded, from shock or fear, or perhaps lost the taste after an illness, but if the cure is to last it must come from your own true desire to stop. Nothing imposed from outside can be really reliable; the first crisis or stress could break your resolve before you realised it.

Savasana, the yoga art of relaxation, removes much of the nervous strain that leads to smoking and there is also a form of self-hypnosis which has helped many smokers to free themselves (see Appendix, page 160).

There is no place for alcohol in a system that puts so much emphasis on physical purification. To intoxicate means to poison – to introduce toxins into the blood – and as we all know, spirits drunk regularly and to excess eventually increase the weight, affect the liver, digestion and nervous system, ruin the complexion and coarsen the features.

Yet it is not always easy to completely avoid alcohol in Western social life. If you are in such a situation and confident that you can take it or leave it alone, that you are really in control of yourself you are not likely to be harmed by an occasional social drink, but if you suspect your own powers of resistance you should completely abstain.

Wine, which is part of the daily diet in some countries, has less alcohol and contains vitamin D, being made from grapes that have ripened in the sun; even so, it should be taken only in moderation and only good wine should be drunk.

One sometimes hears it said that drugs like marihuana are less harmful than alcohol. This may be so but it is a negative statement at best, in view of the damage done by alcohol. It is true that some so-called roadside 'yogis' in India take drugs, but as with the *siddhis* or psychic powers, this has nothing to do with the genuine holy man.

Yoga teaches us that man should be master of himself; 'A king is not one who commands 10,000 slaves but one who commands himself.' To submit will, personality, body and spirit to the domination of so treacherous a master as drugs is completely unacceptable to yoga philosophy.

Chapter Nine

MORE ABOUT YOGA

Apart from the different yogic Paths there are three main kinds of yogis: Ascetic, Tantric and Householder.

We have spoken of Ascetic yogis who live in seclusion, without worldly possessions, observing celibacy and austerities. The Tantric takes the Way of Experience and need not be celibate or vegetarian, or live in seclusion. This Path is dangerous and full of pitfalls without a *guru*, for the teachings of the *Shastras* (the Tantric scriptures) are obscure and often misinterpreted. Tantric schools which concentrate on sex practices as a means of liberation have sometimes been associated with excesses and given the Tantrics a bad name; yet their objective, like all other yogas, is union with God.

The Householder yogi is the one most frequently found in the West. He is usually a *Karma* yogi, living as a married man with his family, working at his job and enjoying life while sincerely following his chosen Path.

It is sometimes difficult for Western minds to understand the real sense of the word 'Path' as used in yoga. We expect paths to be more rigidly defined, their adherents to be confined exclusively to prescribed practices; yet as already explained, yoga has no dogma or ritual. There are no narrow classifications and Paths can merge and overlap. Though a man chooses his Path according to temperament, instinct or intellect he may also follow others to a certain extent. In its widest sense *yoga* could be interpreted as any way of behaving, thinking and living that leads towards God.

The most intellectual and evolved minds are drawn to the higher yogas: *Rajah*, the Royal yoga, which gives complete control of the mind; *Jnani* yoga, the way of knowledge; *Kundalini* yoga, the study of psychic powers and higher faculties, or other esoteric Paths that work through sound, vibration, geometrical forms. Most of the higher Paths demand a way of life that cannot be followed out in the world and are suitable only for disciples living with their *gurus*, in *ashrams* or in seclusion.

Western students may read of these practices but not attempt them. Books never give full instructions and the ancient texts are even more obscure and incomplete. Yoga is meant to be taught directly from teacher to pupil and it is for the *guru* to fill in the gaps and explain the obscurities. Without his help the texts are often meaningless, purposely so to protect the ignorant from tampering with dangerous practices.

Austerities are demanded by the higher yogas in order to conserve all possible energy for achieving *moksa* or Liberation. Nothing must be wasted in unnecessary activity, in emotion, in human relationships, even in speech. Sex energy is also preserved and, like the other energies, transmuted, through yoga techniques, into spiritual and psychic force.

The body must be completely purified before it is ready for higher training. This is done by breath control, diet and techniques for washing out the stomach and intestines.

The higher yogas are lonely paths. The follower of *Jnani* withdraws from all human relationships, subjecting everything to an endless and merciless analysis in his constant search for truth. This Path, which comes naturally to great scholars, philosophers, researchers, is not for the average man.

Nor is *Rajah* yoga. This yogi is also a solitary figure. His Path is difficult and demanding; it embraces other yogas – knowledge, psychic power, mysticism, even *Hatha* yoga, which is sometimes called a stepping-stone to *Rajah* – and is the highest of all.

In *Kundalini* Yoga, the adept works upon the release of the body's latent nervous energy. The techniques used are extremely dangerous and can only be studied under the constant supervision of a *guru*. The subject is complex and abstruse. Briefly, *Kundalini* is the force of nervous or psychic energy in the body. Modern writers have suggested that it is an actual physical nerve but in the ancient texts it is described as a coiled serpent, sleeping at the base of the spine. When the yogi awakens *Kundalini* she rushes up the spinal cord to the brain; in other words Liberation is attained.

On her way she rouses the six *chakras* (nervous plexuses) of the subtle body and as each one is awakened different psychic powers come to life in the yogi. The *chakras* might be compared to a string of electric light bulbs, with the largest one in the head. As *Kundalini* rushes, hissing, up through the spinal canal each light is switched on in turn, ending in a blaze of glory with the biggest light of all, *Brahmachakra*, the Thousand-Petalled Lotus. This is Enlightenment . . . Yoga.

Occasionally people are born with some of the psychic powers released by *Kundalini* – gifted clairvoyants, mind-readers, mediums, possessors of complete photographic memory or phenomenal powers of instant calculation, different kinds of genius – but normally these powers would take thousands of years of evolution to develop.

Kundalini must be a forbidden yoga for the ordinary man. Attempts to rouse her made by the ignorant and untrained end in disaster. An unprepared body cannot take the shock of such a sudden explosion of nervous energy, and permanent illness, insanity and death could result.

It is sometimes said that *Bhakti*, the way of love and devotion, is not a separate Path at all, since devotion should be present in all other yogas. *Bhakti* is the yoga of the great Indian masses, of all devout people whose lives are ruled more by emotion than intellect. It requires no special training or austerities, only a sincere love and desire for union with God. It is the way of religious worship, of loving-kindness towards all men.

Karma yoga, as we know, is the yoga of work and right action, the Path for the Householder, the family man out in the world. A *Karma* yogi tries to live by right action, not only in the direct sense of giving, or helping others but also by refraining from unworthy actions, from cheating, exploiting, taking advantage of those weaker or less businesslike than himself. He works hard and honestly but never at the expense of others and always for the sake of work rather than its rewards.

In the *Bhagavad Gita*, in which *Karma* Yoga is explained, the Lord Krishna tells us that we have the right to work but for the work's sake only, not for its fruits; that desire for rewards should never be the motive in working. This is absolute commonsense. Painters and writers know that work

144

done for its own sake is better than work done only for money; the Paris butcher who arranges his wares in such beautiful patterns, the chef who decorates his cakes with such care both do so for love of their work. They know, by its very nature, that their creation will be destroyed but that does not prevent them from repeating the process, day after day, independent of what they are paid.

Work done for its own sake and work done under pressure, only for rewards, might be compared to a fine Hepplewhite chair and a mass-produced one turned out by factory machines.

This is not to suggest that workers should not be paid. Many of the world's greatest geniuses were obliged to work in order to keep alive; but though, for instance, Mozart composed music for money, you can be sure that while he was doing so it was his work he was thinking of, not how much it would earn. Mozart's life was plagued by financial worries, he died of overwork, so poor that he was buried in a pauper's grave and no one knows where he lies, yet his music shows no hint, no trace of the stresses that haunted him. If he had not been able to turn off his worries and absorb himself in his work, his music would not be, as it is, the very spirit of beauty, untouched by material thought.

As well as detachment in work, the *Karma* yogi also strives to achieve detachment, a sense of non-possession, towards everything. Ordinary householders with responsibilities cannot just give them away and live like ascetic yogis, they must work and provide for their dependents; but they can be detached in their minds, in their attitudes, neither enslaved by material ambition nor possessed by possessions. Possessiveness is the cause of most of our troubles. From earliest infancy we hear the words My ... My ... Mine ... My baby ... My darling child ... My wife ... My country. The passion for owning, which leads to the instinct to fight, could be overcome by yoga.

It is possible to learn to live in normal pleasant surroundings, even surrounded by works of art and material comforts, yet remain detached in the mind; to know that these things are not really important, that they all could be destroyed, that they are toys which must be left behind when

145

we go. Though we constantly hear the saying, 'You can't take it with you', very few people act as though they believed it.

There have been many great *Karma* yogis in the world's history: for instance, St. Francis and Mahatma Gandhi. In Japan there is a community known as Ittoen, The Garden of One Light. It grew round a Japanese spiritual leader, Tenko Nishida, who believed that the only way for man to live in peace was through selfless service and non-possession. The community, which began as a handful of homeless wanderers, is now settled in a beautiful garden village, built by themselves; but Tenko-san never ceased to remind them that though the land had been given by friends and the garden made with their own hands, it was not *theirs*; it was just 'a night's lodging' – a gift from Light, or God, for which they must always give thanks by service to others. This is true *Karma* yoga.

Behind the life of Right Action is a deep spiritual purpose. The word *karma*, meaning *work* or *action* in the ordinary sense, is also the name for the Law of Cause and Effect. This is so closely connected with the doctrine of Reincarnation or Rebirth that they are sometimes described as Twin Doctrines. They cannot be separated; without belief in *karma*, reincarnation loses its purpose and without Reincarnation there would be no *karma*. This doctrine, which is held all through the East, was once a belief of the early Christian church.

Every man, even each nation, has its own *karma*, all subject to the law of cause and effect. We know from everyday life that certain actions, or thoughts, lead inevitably to certain results; in a way it is a form of accepting responsibility for one's own actions; but the doctrine of *karma* teaches that our present life can be influenced by the deeds we have performed in earlier lives, and if they have been bad lives we may have to work out the consequences in this incarnation.

Though this has been called the Law of Moral Retribution, *karma* is less a threatening punishment than a lesson that has to be learnt. If the schoolchild has not done his work today he must come back and do it tomorrow. In each succeeding life we try to learn a little more, to catch up on lessons not learnt yesterday, and to prepare for those ahead. We make our own destiny, our own future lives.

Western critics have said that belief in *karma* creates a negative attitude to life; that if we are already governed by what we did in a previous existence there can be no escape and there is no point in trying. This is not so. Though a belief in *karma* does help develop a sense of acceptance – it explains so much that is otherwise inexplicable, the suffering and injustice endured by harmless people, the extraordinary phenomenon of genius – yet it is neither negative nor harsh. There is always a second chance in the moment of Free Will.

Bad *karma* from past incarnations may confront us with evil situations in this life, but it *cannot force us to act*. We have the choice to accept or reject. If we reject we create good future *karma*, if we succumb we build up more bad *karma*. We can thus influence our future by rejecting temptation and by Right Action, and so work out the mistakes we made in past lives.

When eventually all bad *karma* is gone man becomes free of the Wheel of Reincarnation. He no longer has to go through rebirth on this earth, perhaps into circumstances of misery; his spirit is free to unite for ever with God. He has conquered death.

Sometimes a fully-liberated soul chooses to come back to earth to help and guide humanity, at no matter what cost. There have been very few such great *avatars*: Buddha, Jesus Christ, Mahommed and Lord Krishna are among those honoured in yoga.

Whether or not people accept this doctrine, the path of *Karma* Yoga is a noble one, and as Krishna tells us in the *Gita*, even the attempt that fails is not wasted; it could save man from the terrible wheel of rebirth and death.

Although *Hatha* yoga is the path of bodily strength and control, it is also known as the Three-fold Path, because it trains body, mind and spirit. The *asanas* by which it is so well-known are only one of its 'arms'.

In some ways *Hatha* yoga overlaps *Tantric* yoga, which also cultivates physical health and strength, and it can, as we know, lead on to *Rajah* yoga. The classical texts say that for success in the higher yogas the disciple must first acquire

147

strength and health and a mind completely under control. He must observe intensive purification and not allow his body to deteriorate through lack of exercise. (There is a legend in Japan that Daruma, the first Zen patriarch, sat so long in meditation without moving that his legs wore away.)

There are various ancient Sanscrit texts on *Hatha* yoga but its origins have been lost in time. A romantic legend from China tells that it began at the court of a king. He had fallen deeply in love with a beautiful young woman and was distressed at the thought of her loveliness being ravaged by time. He commanded his wise men to find a way to preserve her youth, and after much study and thought they evolved the system we know as *Hatha* yoga, by which she could hold back old age.

Patanjali, the sage known as the Father of Yoga, listed eight steps to be followed by serious *Hatha* yogis. These are, abstinences; observances; *asanas* (bodily poses); breath control; withdrawal of mind from external influences; concentration; contemplation and identification.

1. The abstinences or *yamas* are:

    Non-violence: To refrain from giving pain in any way, physically or mentally, directly or indirectly, to anyone, even oneself.

    Non-lying: To refrain from acting as well as speaking lies, from direct or indirect untruthfulness.

    Non-stealing: This includes not cheating, not accepting bribes and not condoning stealing by others.

    Chastity: Refraining from lechery and sexual incontinence in thought, word and deed.

    Non-possession: To refrain from possessiveness of any kind towards people, objects, even intangibles, such as power.

2. The observances or *niyamas* are:

    Purity: In body, thought and deed. (Physical purity includes inner and outer bodily cleanliness through bathing, pure diet, and purification of internal organs.)

    Contentment: Acceptance of whatever life brings. Ability to face success or failure, happiness or misery philosophically, without complaint.

    Austerity: Mental and physical. Mental austerities lead to

148

moral strength and courage; they include keeping guard over the tongue and not speaking unkind, angry, hurtful words. Physical austerities, which bring greater tolerance of pain and hardship, include fasting and self-denial of comforts or pleasure.

Devotion to God: Meditation, prayer, study of the scriptures.

Though these *yamas* and *niyamas* may appear at first rather harsh they are really a sound commonsense basis for peaceful and happy living and are, in essence, almost identical with the teachings of Christ. An ascetic yogi must strictly observe them all in every respect but the discipline for householders is not so demanding in certain instances – e.g. celibacy is not enforced – although they should be followed to the best of one's ability.

3. The *asanas*

These are the 84 classical poses by which *Hatha* yoga achieves so many of its effects on the body. Since this book is mainly concerned with them they need not be discussed here, except perhaps to mention the emphasis the ancient texts place on the sitting positions, particularly the Lotus and Adept Poses. One could almost receive the impression that they are the most important of all; but this is not so. The other *asanas* are necessary for keeping the body strong enough to sit for long hours in meditation.

4. Breath Control or *Pranayama*

This is the basis of the whole system, which leads to control of *prana*, of life itself, and to *samadhi*.

5. *Withdrawal*

By learning to turn off the perceptionary senses one can withdraw from the external world without moving the physical body, thus increasing control of mind and senses, a development essential for the last three steps:

6. *Concentration*

Concentration, or fixing the mind upon one point without deviating or wavering, leads to stillness of mind. This is a preliminary for Contemplation.

7. *Contemplation*

In which one dwells upon or contemplates every aspect

of the chosen subject. These two steps, 6 and 7, are sometimes grouped together as one.

8. *Identification*
   This is the higher state of consciousness in which the individual Self or *Atman* is merged with the Universal Self or *Brahman*. This is Liberation of the spirit; yoga.

One sometimes hears it said 'Why go through all these laborious disciplines when *samadhi* can be easily attained through LSD?' The answer is that, apart from the dangers of taking drugs, and assuming that LSD brings only *good* trips, higher consciousness achieved in this way does not seem to have the same value as true spiritual revelation, no matter how similar the actual experience may appear.

Accounts of ecstasy induced by LSD sometimes describe sensations similar to those experienced by yogis: change in breathing tempo; a blinding white light; a force moving up the spine to the brain, as *Kundalini* is said to move; the top of the head exploding, as in the yogic Opening of the Thousand-petalled Lotus to Infinity; ineffable peace, a sense of absolute knowing; Identification.

It all sounds like *samadhi*, if *samadhi* can be described in words. (Words are the tools of thought, an integral part of the mind, and *samadhi* can only come after the mind is completely stilled and all thought suspended.) Yet is it the same? True spiritual illumination has a permanent effect; it changes lives, it does not wear off or die away and become forgotten, whether the actual *samadhi* in which it was attained lasts for short or long periods in our sense of time. One has only to compare LSD addicts with Enlightened holy-men to wonder if *samadhi* reached through the drug can produce fully-realised spirits, or if it only leads to more and more LSD.

Those who have experienced higher consciousness by both yoga and LSD suggest that a fully-trained yogi is more likely to reach *samadhi* through the drug than an ordinary addict whose body is not only unprepared but could also be in poor health; but the question is academic, for who would seek liberation by such a dangerous route when they can attain it safely, in full health and control?

The real way is hard, but is not the training itself of value? The discipline, self-control, perseverence, growth of mental and spiritual strength? Discounting all the still unknown hazards of LSD and how it might damage the brain, such instant results obtained *at will** could have two effects: a cheapening of the experience, or an increased desire for it. Both could be bad, but the latter, when obtained through drugs, could lead to destruction.

The *Upanishads* tell us that when the sages have known the Self they are filled with joy; blessed are they and tranquil of mind, free from passion. This description does not seem to apply to the average LSD addict.

---

*Involuntary *samadhi*, and *satori*, is possible, but since it happens without warning and cannot be recalled at will it can only be regarded as a fluke, a happy accident.

Chapter Ten

PRACTICE GUIDE

To get the most out of your practice, try to remember the following:

1. Whether alone or in a class, concentrate on what you are doing. Five minutes with full concentration are better than half an hour with a wandering mind.
2. Remember that no gesture in yoga is useless or done just for effect; that everything has a purpose.
3. Relaxation and recharging should come before activity, and where possible you should relax and slow down the body between *asanas*.
4. Remember that slow breathing is the key to concentration and to relaxation.
5. Practise in a quiet place where you will not be disturbed, and if possible always the same place, on the same mat. Do not practise in a draught, in front of a fire (because of chills), or for three hours after eating.
6. Always sit straight, when cross-legged, with back and neck in one line.
7. A general knowledge of your own body and its functions gives more intelligent and constructive interest in your practice. It is easier to learn and remember if you know why certain things are done and what their effects will be.
8. Try to learn breathing cycles and *asanas* so you can practise without stopping for reference or to check with the book. This becomes easier as you go on.
9. The best exercise to flex up joints for sitting in the Lotus or Half-lotus Position is the Free Pose (page 87).
10. Remember that in balancing poses, fifty per cent is mental effort.
11. Never force yourself when over-tired. At such times, and also for women who are menstruating, the emphasis should be on relaxing and deep breathing.

12. Never practise to the stage of exhaustion.
13. Be careful. Never strain or force muscles or joints.
14. Remember that pain is a stop signal.
15. Observe the *Cautions and Prohibitions*.
16. Be sure there is no physical reason – e.g. high blood-pressure or disc weakness – that forbids certain poses. If in doubt have a medical check-up before starting.
17. In pregnancy, do not practise without a doctor's approval. In normal cases yoga is excellent so long as nothing is done that might affect the position of the child: stomach contractions, raised poses, headstands and upward stretching are forbidden. Many expectant mothers continue practice till the last moment, gradually eliminating poses that have become uncomfortable. But get medical advice first, in case there is some reason why you should not exercise.
18. Always practise the headstand against a wall, if you are alone, until your balance and confidence are perfect.
19. Proceed slowly. There is no hurry; you are not going for an exam and yoga is non-competitive.
20. Do not be easily discouraged. Regard every difficulty as a challenge to be overcome.
21. Remember that for full achievement you must use the three powers: power of breath, power of bodily position and power of concentration.
22. In using this book study all illustrations carefully and *read the whole text*.

SUGGESTED PRACTICE FOR THOSE WITH VARYING AMOUNTS OF FREE TIME

Whenever possible, include *Savasana*, even if the only time is after getting into bed at night.

A.   *For those with minimum time*

On getting out of bed: Limbering up; forward stretching and waistline exercises; Vigorous recharging cycle.
Under the shower, or in bathroom: *Uddiyana* or *Nauli*.

B. *Alternative minimum time*
On getting out of bed (or if this is not possible, whenever you can): *Surya Namaskar* – Greeting to the Rising Sun.

C. *With a little extra time during the day*
Practice A and/or B on getting up; during the day add Spinal Twist and Shoulderstand. Before bedtime, *Savasana*.

D. *If time allows*
Practice A, and/or B, plus C, and add: Additional preliminary exercises; Shoulderstand; Pose of Tranquillity; Arch gesture; Spinal Twist; and Headstand, if being practised.

E. *With more time available*
Practice A, and/or B, plus C, D and the following: Pacifying Breaths; Archer; Sideways Swing; Supine Pelvic; one Raised Pose.

F. *With more time still*
Practice A, B, plus C, D, E, and the following: Half-shoulderstand; one Balancing pose; two forward-stretching variations of Arch Gesture; *Bhastrica*.

G. *With unlimited time*
Full hour's practice, including exercises for eyes, head and neck and mental exercises, plus quiet breathing.

The exercises and *asanas* listed in the following pages are given as *suggested guides*, not necessarily to be followed slavishly. Learn to build your own lesson or practice, but try to follow the general order or sequence as shown in this book.

There is a timetable for each day of the week. Number 1 is the lesson in the main text of the book (Monday practice).

If possible, include a mental exercise every day. For instance, you could work on the Seven Fears, taking a different one for each day of the week.

NUMBER 2
TUESDAY PRACTICE

Savasana
Limbering up exercises
Quiet Recharging Cycle
Exercises for chest, waistline, legs
Pacifying Cycle
Greeting to the Rising Sun
Pose of a Fish
Shoulderstand
Half-shoulderstand
Pose of Tranquillity
Balancing Shoulderstand
Cobra pose – with head back; with chin held in
Pose of a Locust
Bow Pose
Spinal massage
In cross-legged pose: Slow breathing
Mental Exercise: Creating a Flower
Head, neck, eye exercises
4 digestive movements
Uddiyana, sitting position
Arch Gesture *plus* 2 variations
Pose of a Star
Splits pose
Head to Knee pose – sitting
Pose of an Archer
Spinal Twist
Sideways Swing
Pose of a Camel
Pose of a Child
Supine Pelvic
Pose of a Bird
Savasana
Shaking of limbs
Headstand

NUMBER 3
WEDNESDAY PRACTICE

Savasana
Limbering up
Great Physical Breath of a Yogi
Slow Movements, for stomach muscles
Uddiyana and/or *Nauli* – standing
Pacifying Cycle
Shoulderstand
Half-shoulderstand
Pose of Tranquillity
Balancing Shoulderstand
Breathing in Sleeping Positions
Cobra Pose; both variations
Half-Locust Pose
Pose of a Locust
Spinal Massage
In cross-legged pose: Easy Pose or Pose of an Adept
Mental Exercise: Universal Goodness
Head, Neck, Eye exercises
Pose of a Lion
Arch Gesture and two variations
Pose of a Star
Splits Pose
Head-to-Knee – sitting
Pose of an Archer
Variation of Archer Pose
Sideways Swing
Spinal Twist
Pose of a Cat
Supine Pelvic Pose
Pose of a Child
Pose of Eight Curves
Savasana
Shaking of limbs
Headstand

RELAX BETWEEN POSES

NUMBER 4
THURSDAY PRACTICE
Savasana
Limbering up
Recharging Cycle
Preliminary exercises: Slow Movements for arms, shoulders, bust
Greeting to the Rising Sun
Shoulderstand
Half-shoulderstand
Pose of Tranquillity
Balancing Shoulderstand
Plough Pose
Advasana
Cobra Pose: both variations
Locust Pose
Bow Pose
Spinal Massage
In cross-legged pose: Head, neck, eye exercises
In Pose of a Hero: Mental exercise; Development of Inner Strength
Arch Gesture and two variations
Head-to-Knee Pose – sitting
Pose of an Archer
Variation of Archer Pose
Little Twist
Sideways Swing
Spinal Twist
Pose of a Child
Pose of a Hare
Supine Pelvic Pose
Pose of a Raven
Uddiyana – standing position
Savasana
Shaking limbs
Headstand

NUMBER 5
FRIDAY PRACTICE
Savasana
Limbering up
Quiet Recharging Cycle
Rocking – Spinal massage
Pose of a Tree
Pose of an Eagle
Pose of a Frog
Shoulderstand
Half-shoulderstand
Pose of Tranquillity
Balancing Shoulderstand
Half-Wheel Pose
Angular Pose
In cross-legged pose: Facial exercises; Head, neck and eye exercises
Mental Exercise: I am Master of Myself
Uddiyana – sitting position
Head of a Cow Pose
Arch Gesture and two variations
Pose of a Star
Splits Pose
Head-to-Knee Pose – sitting
Pose of an Archer
Sideways Swing
Spinal Twist
Solar plexus Pose
Pose of a Bird
Pose of a Cat
Pose of a Child
Supine Pelvic Pose
Savasana
Shaking limbs
Headstand

RELAX BETWEEN POSES

NUMBER 6
SATURDAY PRACTICE
Savasana
Limbering up
Recharging Cycle
Preliminary exercises
Pacifying Cycle
Head-to-Knee – standing
Pose of an Eagle
Uddiyana and/or *Nauli* –
  standing
Plough Pose
Shoulderstand
Half-shoulderstand
Pose of Tranquillity
Balancing Shoulderstand
Breathing in Sleeping
  positions
Pose of a Cobra: two
  variations
Half-Locust Pose
Pose of a Locust
Pose of a Bow
Spinal Massage
Cross-legged poses: Adept;
  Half-Lotus; Lotus
  position
In cross-legged position:
  Head, neck, eye exercises
Mental Exercise: I am
  Stronger than Fear
Solar plexus Pose
Angular Pose
Arch Gesture and two
  variations
Pose of an Archer
Sideways Swing
Spinal Twist
Pose of a Camel
Pose of a Child

Supine Pelvic Pose
Pose of a Hare
Inverted Bird Pose
Savasana
Headstand

RELAX BETWEEN POSES

NUMBER 7
SUNDAY PRACTICE
Savasana
Limbering up
Quiet Recharging Cycle
Preliminary exercises and
    Slow Movements
Greeting to the Rising Sun
Breath of Circulating Life
    Force
Shoulderstand
Half Shoulderstand
Pose of Tranquillity
Balancing Shoulderstand
Modified Fish Pose
Diamond Pose
In cross-legged pose: Slow
    breathing
Mental exercise: Protective
    Cocoon
Head, neck, eye exercises
4 movements for digestive
    organs
Uddiyana and/or *Nauli* –
    sitting
Pose of Eight Curves
Arch Gesture and two
    variations
Pose of a Star
Splits Pose
Head-to-Knee – sitting pose
Pose of an Archer
Variation of Archer Pose
Little Twist
Sideways Swing
Spinal Twist
Cobra Pose: two variations
Bow Pose
Supine Pelvic Pose
Pose of a Child

Inverted Bird Pose
Savasana
Shaking of limbs
Headstand

RELAX BETWEEN POSES

FOR FURTHER READING

Students who are really interested will not be content with beginners' books such as this; they will want to know more about the different yogas and probably about *Hatha* yoga in particular.

The following books are suggested as a start. As the student reads more widely he will find for himself other references to follow up.

For general use:
*Yoga and Health,** by Yesudian and Elisabeth Haich.
Yoga for the Western World, by Sir Paul Dukes.
Any other yoga books by Sir Paul Dukes.
Any books on yoga by Indra Devi.
*Yoga for Women**
*Yoga over Forty**
Yoga Breathing⎬ by Michael Volin and Nancy Phelan.
*Sex and Yoga**
Any books on yoga by Ramacharaka.

More advanced:
*Hatha Yoga,** by Theos Bernard.
Yoga: the method of Reintegration, by Alain Danielou.
The Mysterious Kundalini, by Dr V. Rele.
*Yoga,** by Ernest Wood.

Background reading:
*The Upanishads.**
*The Bhagavad Gita.**
*A Search in Secret India,** by Paul Brunton.
The Hidden teaching behind Yoga, by Paul Brunton.
*Maharishi Ramana and the Path of Self Knowledge,** by A. Osborne.

*Available in paperback.

APPENDIX

SMOKING
(Quoted from: *Yoga over Forty* by Michael Volin and Nancy Phelan)

Start with meditation on the subject of smoking.

1. Sit cross-legged in a secluded place, preferably in the open, and establish deep breathing. Enjoy every moment of it, concentrating on the thought of the purity of the air, the pleasure of inhaling it, the delicate tissues of the lungs and how easily they can be damaged.

2. Promise yourself that you will stop smoking just for three days, which is not really hard to do, and tell yourself that you are strong enough to do it.

3. Tell yourself that you will lose self-respect if you do not fulfil this promise, and encourage yourself by the thought that after three days of abstaining the backbone of the habit will be broken.

4. The next time you smoke, destroy your psychological pleasure by thinking negatively about smoking (the main pleasure of smoking is psychological) and you will find that you have lost your craving. To think negatively in this instance means to dwell upon all the depressing consequences, the suffering and misery of lung cancer, of any lung damage, upon the humiliating position of being dependent on tobacco, even on the expense of your bad habit.

5. To further strengthen your morale and determination, think positively about yourself and your character; how much better your feel in being really master of yourself. Remember the old proverb: 'A master is not one who commands ten thousand slaves, it is one who is master of himself.'